SCARED DAD FEEDING

How My Daughter's Anorexia Took Me to Hell, and My Guidebook for How I Got Back

Kevin E. Olmsted

Scareddadfeeding.com
https://www.linkedin.com/in/kevinolmsted/

ISBN 979-8-9852637-0-1 print
ISBN 979-8-9852637-2-5 ebook
Library of Congress Control Number: 2022908409
Edited by Dr. Heather Wood
Interior design by Val Sherer, Personalized Publishing Services

Contents

Introduction

This book is about how my wife and I accompanied our daughter on her trip to hell with anorexia. It is a book about how we navigated a foreign and unheard-of world. It is a book about how we failed, about what we learned, about what we figured out and are still figuring out, and finally about how we persevered. It is just our story; it is just our perspective. And though parts of it are meant to be prescriptive, not all of the advice will apply to everyone. I hope you can either relate to parts of our story or learn a trick that helps you. We are not experts, nor do we mean to preach a method. We will suggest a few ideas and express a few opinions that some folks may disagree with. But our intention is to share our experience, and to share our path.

This book is also about how we treated our daughter and facilitated her recovery from anorexia. My wife, Tina, and I have been together for over 30 years. We are partners, we are best friends, and we are soul mates. The reason I am doing the writing and emphasizing the father point of view (which will partially be explained in Chapter 7) is because of how our two careers went in different directions. I have been in wine sales for 23 years, and I have mastered the flexible schedule. *The 4-Hour Workweek* is one of my favorite books. In the last seven years, I have stepped in to handle more of the house and kid duties because I could, and because our teenagers and their lives demanded it. Tina has always worked a corporate job, with a hefty commute, and she has also in recent years achieved a very high level of responsibility. So, when our daughter got sick, and we started our slog through hell, my career coincidentally came to a natural "pause point" that we decided to exploit. I immediately dropped any care I had for my career path or my title so that I could jump in and do all of the day-to-day care for our daughter. This was going to be the most important thing I could do as a parent, and no amount of wine sales mattered in comparison.

As the primary author, I am not a doctor nor a therapist, and I have no formal training with eating disorders. I base this whole book on my research, my interviews, and my experiences. I am not an authority, I am just a parent. And uniquely, I am just a dad. I have not seen much from fathers about their experiences with their kids' eating disorders, yet I know many are struggling just as much as mothers. Also, my daughter's eating disorder is anorexia nervosa, which is mostly based on food restriction and avoidance. Other prominent eating disorders, such as bulimia nervosa, binge/purge and ARFID (Avoidant Restrictive Food Intake Disorder) do share certain traits with anorexia, but they are all unique. I do not mean to avoid discussing these other disorders, but the authenticity of our story is based only on our experience with anorexia.

There is obviously some madness to the method by which I organized the chapters in this book. I intended many of them to be somewhat like silos unto themselves. I found that it is ok if some ideas or topics just plop down in the middle of nowhere. My normal instinct is usually to "tell the story," bullet point the timeline, and go through it all in a linear manner. But that would almost take away from the fun of telling each piece separately. Most folks in the eating disorder community who read this book will already know the story. Hell, by virtue of the fact that they are reading this, they have probably already *lived* the story. If you are new to our community, I am horrifically sorry to welcome you. But you will all understand my journey by the end of the book.

Finally, it was recommended to me that I not use my daughter's name, and instead I should give her a pseudonym. For three of the most powerful reasons I can think of, I will call her "M". It is the first initial in English of one of her grandmothers, and the middle initial of the same name, but in Danish, of her other grandmother. Finally, her mother's Danish middle name also starts with M. The blood of these three strong and incredible women run through her, and it is this power that makes her the hero of this story.

To M:
We love you,
and we can't give you enough of that.

Chapter 0
You Can Do This, Dads

You all should query "Anorexia" in the book section of Amazon. You know, the place where you bought this book. When the results pop up, just scroll through the first few pages, and make a mental note of the first name of most of the authors. Those names are going to be female names. And to go one step further, see about whom most of the memoirs are written. Again, I'm going to bet you that those are female names.

This is just one small metric to highlight a major tenet of this book. The dominant voices in literature, in chat groups, and in online posts that speak about eating disorders are coming from women. Those voices are coming from Mothers about their daughters, and those voices are coming from women who are describing their experiences as little girls. The perspective of men, of fathers, and of boys is glaringly absent from the journey and struggle and discussion of eating disorders. And most often when a man does weigh in with a book, he is usually a doctor or a professor writing from a clinical or an academic perspective.

I have been a father for over 20 years. I have seen

way too many other fathers leave most of the parenting to their wives. I have seen way too many fathers tune out their kids. Parenting takes two people, and supporting the treatment and recovery of a child suffering from a mental disorder will be twice as effective when there are two parents.

Dads, I am not going to belabor this point, because I know you get it. You may pretend not to, or you may just want to ignore it. But here's the truth. If your kid, either your son or your daughter, is struggling with an eating disorder, you need to be fully involved. Your kid needs both you and your wife (assuming, of course, you are both together and/or around). Your kid is going through the most terrifying experience of their life, and if both parents are standing by to help them, their chances for recovery are much greater.

There are plenty of fathers out there who are very involved with their kids, but even they know that this appeal is valid and needs to be said. This is meant to be positive and encouraging. Dads are capable of amazing things when it comes to parenting, and there is no greater accomplishment than helping to save the life of your kid.

Lock in, Dads. You can do this.

Chapter 1
Abandon All Hope

The fear and pain and terror of eating disorders are debilitating and paralyzing. Every part of your mind, your feelings, your outlook and your spirit become compromised. You live in a vacuum where hope and horizon do not exist. Initially, this all comes out of nowhere and hits you like a brick. As you slide down into this morass, you thrash about trying to learn where you are and why this is happening, all while the mortality clock is ticking. And even when you bottom out and learn what's going on, where you are, how bad things have become, and how impossible it is to climb back out, all those oppressive and confining feelings have to be ignored if you have any chance of survival or success. And while it would be sound to assume that I am talking about those who suffer from eating disorders, I am actually talking about the folks who treat the suffering. I'm talking about the parent of a kid who cannot eat because of a raging mental disorder that is trying to kill her. I'm talking about me.

The first time these feelings hit me was in June of 2019. M, my daughter, was just finishing her freshman year of high school, and she was finding success across most of her endeavors. Her older brother was a senior at the same school, and even he admitted that she was really fitting in and standing out. She took a zero period, meaning that she was up and out early, and also that she took seven classes in her first year, yet earned a place on the honor roll with a 3.7 grade point average. She was popular and part of a big social group. She was picking up followers on social media. She was asked to homecoming, and then had a few boys from various schools asking her out. Hell, I had other parents, parents of her friends, take me aside and tell me she was a baller.

The previous fall, she tried out for and made the freshman girls' soccer team, which was no small feat considering that the school's varsity girls' soccer team regularly competed for league and state championships. That program was for elite athletes, but we also live in a community full of high-achieving parents, competitive sports programs, and Type A kids. M was a starter the whole season and her speed up front made her stand out as other teams had to mark her. Overlapping with the end of the soccer season, she went straight over to a starting position on the junior varsity girl's lacrosse team. Here again, she played at a very high level, leading the team in ground balls, assists, shots on goal, and was second in goals scored. Her coaches awarded her MVP of the midline at the end of the year and predicted that she would make the varsity team as a sophomore.

Within a week of lacrosse ending, we saw her doctor about a pain in her hip, who referred us to an orthopedic surgeon. After the exam and an MRI, it turned out that a plate on her left hip bone had still not finished growing, and it was causing a debilitating tissue bruise that made running, and sometimes walking, hurt. So, we went to physical therapy two times a week for the eight weeks leading up to the end of school and the start of summer. And she was no longer allowed to run or exercise.

This is where the train started to go off the rails.

All the ways in which I have described M are the same behaviors of kids with a typical eating disorder (ED) profile. These kids are high achievers in sports, social activities, and academics. They are rule-followers and people-pleasers. They are Type A and hyper-focused. And then all, or some, of these successes come up against a roadblock like an injury, and these innocent children, carrying all this focus and drive, can no longer hold back the mental disorder that has been waiting for an opening to strike.

So, in June 2019, I was sitting on our back patio in the middle of the afternoon, hiding in the shade of an umbrella, and looked up when I heard the back door open. M was walking toward the pool, towel over her shoulder and huge aviator sunglasses covering half her face. It was summer, it was hot, and she had on a bikini. It barely clung to her shriveled shell of a body. At first, I saw M's hip bone sticking out because her suit bottoms were hanging onto them to defy gravity. Then I noticed her shoulder bones were like coat hangers keeping up her suit top. Next, she leaned over to spread out her towel, and her arched backbone stuck out of her pale skin like a dinosaur skeleton. Not long before this, I had happily watched her strong and athletic body run around the lacrosse field. But this day, I was shocked and nauseous at the sight of her. This was also when the fear set in. I didn't know what of, but I was upside down. And it wasn't just her appearance, it was her deep yet quiet voice, it was the cold and dark look in her eyes. It was her indifference to my inquiries about her weight, and then about her eating, and then about her obsession with weird water concoctions, and then about her getting back into exercising even though she hadn't been cleared by the doctor. She wasn't 'she' anymore, she was pushing back on anything I said and was retreating and running away from our relationship. And suddenly I didn't know her.

Just two months earlier, I was driving carpool for her lacrosse team. She was hugging me after games. We were doing our normal post-game breakdown of her performance, usually with a lot of dark humor, but really evaluating what was good and bad. We were stopping for food or making stuff together in the kitchen at home. We were best friends back then. But not anymore.

For the next month, my fear became a constant state of anxiety as M continued to refuse to eat or acknowledge that there was anything wrong with her. The only idea I came up with was to get her into her pediatrician for a fall sports physical. Maybe the doctor would see the signs and get M some medical help and be the one to stop this madness. Unfortunately, as I will discuss in greater detail later, the pediatrician turned out to not be the person we needed to see. She was like many physicians, who are not trained to recognize or diagnose eating disorders, and this lack of experience led her to simply refer M to a dietician. Here again, while the dietician gave us fabulous information about food, there was no real treatment for the mental disorder that was infecting M's mind.

Our lost and meandering journey went on through July, all the while I stupidly let her play club lacrosse tournaments in Illinois and Oregon... oh, I paid to travel around the country with her while she was a whisper of her former self. I thought I was forcing her to eat, but I was delusional. She was so far gone, I had no ability to affect her behavior. I had nothing. I was so angry, and while I thought I was angry at her, I was angry at myself. What the fuck was I doing? She was physically melting away in front of my eyes, and she was becoming so bitter and dismissive.

The fear in me went up a level on Saturday, July 27th. The day before, we had somehow gotten in to see a psychologist who worked with eating disorder patients... but we still didn't say "eating disorder." We didn't think it. We didn't know it. The enormity of anorexia was just about to hit us like a sucker punch. Like any surprise trauma life, you don't know you've been sucker punched in the face until you're lying on the ground staring up at the asshole who did it. In this case, the asshole was the demon, was the eating disorder everyone calls "ED," was anorexia trying to kill my daughter.

The psychologist saw M for an hour late on a Friday. After we left, she called the most preeminent eating disorder physician in the area, Dr. Sue Knight, and begged to have M seen the next morning. Ironically, we had an appointment with Dr. Knight for later in

August, but what the psychologist saw in M was classic anorexia that was becoming medically dangerous.

When we arrived at Dr. Knight's office on that Saturday morning, it was very quiet, and we were the first people there. Right away the nurses took M into the back, where they took a urine sample, and then laid M down to begin taking vitals. Tina and I waited in a separate room, not knowing what to expect or why this would be any different from M's pediatrician appointment.

After a while, Dr. Knight called us in to talk without M. She informed us the situation with M was dire and she needed immediate medical attention. Dr. Knight said M's weight was 88 pounds, down from 120+ in April. Her resting heart rate was 41. (She would go on to have an overnight heart rate in the 30s.) Her orthostatia was on the dangerous end of the spectrum: the change in her heart rate from lying down to standing up was +60. Her blood pressure barely registered.

These vital signs were alarming and Dr. Knight recommended M be admitted to an in-patient treatment center immediately. She then told us about the treatment program at Stanford Hospital that could help M, because it is specifically designed to save the health and lives of people whose vital signs are this poor. The program stops the decline in weight and heart strength, starts the refeeding, monitors the vitals, and gets the kids medically stable. Dr. Knight had already called Stanford and they confirmed that a bed was available. It was now time to talk to M. This was the moment, we were later told by our psychologist, that M was about to slip under the surface of quicksand, and we only had one rope left to throw at her.

M came back into the room, sitting between us while Dr. Knight explained her medical situation. She told M that she was vastly underweight, that she was not healthy, that her condition was life-threatening, and that she needed immediate help. M started to cry, but she didn't protest. She knew. She also felt very deeply and secretly the first twinge of relief in months. (M told us much later that she had passed out in our shower the night before this appointment.) She knew something had to break. So, we took her to Stanford Hospital to save her life.

The hospital is about an hour drive from our house, and while I don't remember if or what we talked about, I do remember the music. M had her phone plugged into the car stereo, and was playing all her comfort songs, songs she would blast repeatedly with her friends, or after games. One Direction. Five Seconds of Summer. Soldier Boy. I can remember thinking I could hear her thoughts, feel her emotions as she laid her cheek on the back seat window looking at the side of the road while we drove. Crying.

I think that maybe the difference between fear and scared is a matter of sequence. Fear is when you may not know, you're unsure, it's not defined what's up. Scared is when the shit shows up and you see it. The monster no longer *might* live under your bed or in the closet, it busts the fuck out like Sully and bares its teeth with a roar.

You are scared.

We got to Stanford Hospital, went up to the 4th

floor, rang the bell and were let into the ward. M was immediately taken to her room to get hooked up to a heart monitor and set up in her bed. Tina and I were at the nurse's station doing intake paperwork, getting some kind of introduction, confirming insurance. Then it hit me. I never knew what path we were on. I never knew I had been walking on railroad tracks in the dark with my earbuds in, unable to hear the approaching train. I just happened to step off the tracks for a minute, and the freight rumbled by…the concussive wave of air blasting me as a warning or a reminder of what we barely avoided. My daughter could have died within a week if we hadn't come to the hospital.

This is scary shit.

A couple of days into this first hospital stay, M was no longer confined to bedrest and was allowed to move around in a wheelchair. I wheeled her around as much of the 4th floor as I could find. In the most relaxed and secluded manner, she told me she was relieved to be in the hospital. She didn't have to make decisions or fight her demon, she just had to obey. She just had to eat. It was a stress relief for her. Hearing and knowing that was cathartic for me, but at the same time kind of retroactively stressful. *She* always knew she wanted relief from the demon, but *we* never knew.

Holy shit, I am scared of this demon.

You have to know that hospitalization is not about treating or curing an eating disorder. This is a MASH unit where they triage the worst, do the hard work to get patients stabilized, and then get these folks healthy enough to go back to real treatment. You are released from hospitalization once you no longer need hospitalization. Your vitals (weight, resting heart rate, orthostatia, blood pressure) need to be back in the black, not in the red. After a week in the hospital, and after all the consultation from the crew of eating disorder experts on staff, we were then faced with her discharge. Time for next steps. Time to treat her out there in the real world. But how? Does she go away full-time to a residential facility? Does she attend PHP (Partial Hospitalization Program) or IOP (Intensive Outpatient Program)? Do we all use Family-Based Treatment (FBT)… who's your treatment team?

This is next-level scared.

During one of our many sessions with M and the hospital's in-house psychologist, I stupidly got both M and myself really worked up. The psychologist outlined to us in vague terms a description of Family-Based Treatment (FBT), which was one method of living with and feeding M upon release. This included one of us eating every meal with M and supervising her afterward to ensure that no food was hidden or purged. I then made some insensitive, though I thought funny, comment about how M and I would be having lunch at school together for the next year in the parking lot and how fun it would be.

Wrong thing to say.

Fuck, M lost it. She went off on me and started crying. Tina and I had to leave. It took me an hour or so to calm down and realize M's fear, her anxiety, and her acceptance of this new reality. I texted her a soul-bearing note about my insensitivity, my stupidity, and my love for her. It took a while, but she finally responded and acknowledged it. Unspoken, we both knew we had a long road to go.

I had just gotten my daughter stabilized in the hospital and now they were sending me home. It was like when she was a newborn and they let me go. And I was, like, WTF? I have to leave and do this on my own? It was the same kind of feeling this time, but way worse. I was terrified of her. Tina and I had committed to treating her at home via FBT. Basically, no institutions, we would do it as a family. She answers to us and not any doctors.

I was scared to run a feeding schedule for a girl I just learned has a mental disorder with the highest mortality rate of any mental disorder. I was scared of the fights she would put up. I was scared that she would run away, and I would have to run after her. I was scared she would hurt herself or hurt us or hurt our animals. I was scared that I would have to put up a bigger fight and hold her accountable and go to war for three hours over a plate of food. I was terrified about battling with my little girl, my best friend from soccer and lacrosse games, the kid whose smile and laugh can bring me to my knees. I would have to suit up and beat back the beast in her, but I would only see her. And it will go on for years, with no guarantee that we would make progress.

I'm fucked.

Then there's the fear of admitting your daughter to a residential facility when your first attempt at FBT fails. Or the fear of her getting a one-day pass to come home from that residential care. Or when she gets out of residential care and comes home for good. Or when you get her into PHP, and every day that you pick her up.

All of this nauseating terror ramped up around Thanksgiving 2019. M had been out of residential treatment and attending an outpatient (PHP) program for 45 days. But starting in mid-November, both the head therapist and the dietician at PHP had been telling me that M was stalling out, losing weight, that she needed "another level of care." This diagnosis and recommendation was also coming from Dr. Knight who was monitoring M's vitals weekly. Coincidentally, Tina had a work trip to Denver in mid-November, where she visited the Eating Recovery Center (ERC), one of the best eating disorder treatment program facilities in the country. This would be a bigger residential program than the one M had already lived in, followed by a step-down PHP program, all the while involving the parents. I live in Northern California, so a lot of travel is looming. Hell, how would we even get M on the initial flight out there? When Tina left ERC, she put M on the waiting list for a room. I was starting to plan on flying to Denver every weekend throughout the holidays and into the New Year. Another missed semester of school would mean M would never have her sophomore year. This made me sad for M, thinking of all the things she would miss out on and the potential effect on her college admissions opportunities.

On the Friday before Thanksgiving, Tina and I went to M's PHP facility for our weekly family therapy session. We brought up to M that admitting her to ERC Denver was an option to increase her level of treatment and get her moving toward recovery. Very soon after that, M stormed out of the room.

Tina and I, as well as the PHP psychologist and dietician, followed M and found her on the floor of the waiting room. She was sitting, crammed between a couch and a side table. Her knees were bent up, her arms were wrapped around them, her head was down, and she was crying. We all found spots on the floor around the furniture and sat down with her. I asked her how we could help and what we could do to make her feel safe or happy. She was shaking and breathing hard, she was having trouble speaking. She whispered that she didn't want to fail, that she wanted to find recovery. She said she knew her weight was going back down, and that she was still hiding and restricting food. She said the voice of the demon in her head was too strong for her and that she was terrified that she would never have the strength to resist or seek recovery. And then, out of nowhere, in the quiet and tense air of that waiting room, she asked for the most mature and unseen option I could have predicted: could we could check her back into Stanford Hospital right then? Could she reset, start over, could she please get some un-assailable structure to get her back on track? She said that she didn't want to go to back into a residential facility, and she specifically did not want to go to Denver to ERC. She admitted that she was slipping and in trouble. She told us that she was scared.

She spent five more days in the hospital this second time. What made those days worse than the first hospital visit was what Tina suggested we needed to do going forward. Tina had been reading and analyzing the merits of continued reliance on institutionalized treatments versus Family Based Treatment (FBT). Homeschooling her recovery, so to speak. Battling the beast not only on the home turf, but in the place where M had to eventually come back. This was the first time I ever had shortness of breath and dizziness and a racing heart. I was thinking about managing her anorexia and battling the demon at home, being the only person to bar the door, being the foe to her disorder. This was the fear of not knowing how bad it was going to be and scared because I'd seen some of it before.

When she was discharged from the hospital, we told M that we were pulling her out of PHP and were going to stay home full-time to treat her, along with the help of an FBT therapist. Tina was going to take FMLA (Family Medical Leave Act) from work, and I was going to just punt on wine sales for a while. M shut down all communications with us, and she became very cold and angry. Dark. Evil. That night, the day she got out of the hospital, she ran away. It was dark, it was raining, and we were out of town in a rental house for the long holiday weekend. That was the first time I had cried in years. I grabbed Tina and sobbed. I was panicking, I was imagining the worst scenarios, I was terrified of who or what M was becoming. We called in both the city police and county sheriff. They didn't find her, but M came walking back in the door on her own a couple of hours later. She was wet and cold and shivering, but she had a stone-cold countenance on her face. She said she ran away to make us scared.

The first night we got back from Thanksgiving break, we may have been in our home, but we were really in the boxing ring. The battle was about to start. M ate her dinner with very little resistance, but when we enforced the night snack, she started fighting back. She screamed that she would never eat night snack, that she didn't have to obey us, and that she hated everything about us. She told us to fuck off, and then she started trying to lock herself in rooms around the house. We had to stay calm and keep pushing all five of those Ritz crackers, no matter what. And when I went into the kitchen to get more crackers because M had flushed the first batch down the toilet, I heard the front door open and slam shut. It was the first of a few times I had to run after her through the streets of our neighborhood. This time, I caught her a few houses away in the street. In the rain. While I kept my cool, each time it ended with me hugging her hard and bringing her down to a sitting position in the street. Just to calm her down, to stop her from going, but also to show her that I was serious. No, to show the demon that I was serious about this battle and that I would not be dissuaded from pursuing this treatment and getting my daughter re-fed. You want to take my daughter for a joy ride? Fuck you. I'm stronger. And when she turned around and put on a show about being mad and was stomping back toward the house, I was cool with that. The demon knew it lost that round.

Six weeks into our second attempt at FBT, we hit a really bad spot. I'm foggy on which shitstorm it was. I think it was the second time we called the cops on her, but the result was the proclamation that may have changed my life forever. M told Tina and me, in a much longer and profanity-laden speech, that if we thought we could control or hurt or change her, then she would do worse to us in return. Because we had taken away so much away from her (freedom and control), she was going to take even more away from us. She was going to hurt herself. She was going to hurt us. She was going to hurt the dogs. She was going to hurt other people. And she was going to disappear. She was going back down the rabbit hole to hell to live skinny forever.

Chapter 2
Head Games

Who would think that eating would be hard? It's beyond instinctive to acknowledge hunger and feed yourself. A baby's first cry is for food. Our stomachs rumble and we feel nauseous when they are hollow. We get a headache from low blood sugar when we don't eat enough. Our greatest sense of desire and craving comes from wanting specific foods. Hunger is instigated by smells, by sight, even by memory. Hunger can drive you to consume beyond what your body needs, because hunger is a strong motivator. A certain dish in Italy or Peru or Cleveland will make you book plane tickets. Wanting to eat will instigate the process of planning for, shopping for, and prepping for a dinner party with friends because you want to make a certain dish that tastes great. Consuming food can release endorphins and bring about calm and happiness. Convincing yourself to have a little extra treat after a meal, in the form of a dessert, can make you giggle against guilt. Eating is the fundamental engine to a multi-billion dollar, worldwide industry of restaurants and food trucks and cooking shows and farmers markets and kitchen gadgets and BBQs and blogs.

Who the fuck doesn't want to eat food?

But eating disorders are mental disorders. This is because the brain of someone with an eating disorder is giving bad orders to that person, orders that are antithetical to the instincts, good health and well-being of that person. This mental disease, this demon voice inside a person's head is pushing behavior that can and will kill that person. Eating disorders have the highest mortality rate of any mental disorder, because someone with an eating disorder either starves themselves to death or commits suicide because the anxiety and terror become too much to handle.

Please take a moment and think about these two paragraphs. Our most instinctive, pleasurable and satisfying behavior can be fodder for the deadliest mental disease ever diagnosed. The act and process that keeps us alive on a daily basis can be turned around to make us want to kill ourselves.

Eating disorders have a chicken and egg profile when you go looking for their origins or causes. On one hand, they start as a psychological disorder of the brain that pushes certain thoughts and emotions to the forefront, and those in turn lead the patient to take certain actions. Those actions snowball into patterns of behavior that avoid, restrict, hide, and purge food. On the other hand, a person may begin to restrict and avoid eating to lose weight, behaviors that unknowingly get pushed too far, which in turn create a sense of starvation and euphoria and alter the state of the mind. The disordered thinking germinates and then reinforces the behavior. Great, right? Regardless of how it starts, there are both psychological and physiological patterns that have to be addressed and corrected. I will refer to this general dynamic throughout the book as "state vs. weight." The strength or state of mind that is being compromised by the psychologically disordered thinking vs. the physiological actions of eating, gaining and keeping up weight.

An ED patient suffers greatly from "weight" issues by being underfed, or by having a low heart rate, or by having their organs fail or by having their teeth fall out. But the "state" issues inside the mind of the child with an eating disorder are what drives all of the pain and fear and suffering. The state of mind is the command center and the reactor core on the Death Star, the one spot where you have to place your proton torpedo shot if you are going to blow this thing up. Therapy for this state of mind comes in many forms and has to be done in phases. For example, very early on when a patient is vastly underfed and malnourished and is trying to get blood pressure and heart rate back up, or defecate for the first time in a month, or be even able to absorb 1000 calories into a shrunken stomach, there is very little mental clarity to work with. Sobriety is a long way off, and the demon still rules the mind with twisted and disordered commands. Any kind of therapy here should simply be aimed at facilitating the act of eating. Whether with carrot or stick, the goal is to start the refeeding process in order to gain enough strength of body so that there develops enough strength of mind to receive therapy.

Even as the body gets stronger and the mind starts to accept the concept that eating is in its best interest, the disordered thinking will throw everything at a therapist who is trying to help. "Let's talk about your image of your body," says the therapist. "I fucking hate my body, I can feel my thighs getting bigger," says the demon via the patient. "Where do you want to be in a year?" "I'll be nowhere! I'm never getting better, this disease goes on for, like, 5-10 years. You told me that! I'll never go back to school, I have no friends left, I'll never play sports. Why should I even care or try?" Therapy for the mind at this point is pick and shovel work, and any inch that is won after a week can easily be erased in a second.

The approach that works best for us, one that treats both state of mind and weight gain, is the FBT model, standing for Family Based Treatment. This is done at home, by the parents, with guidance from an FBT therapist. It is based on exposure and openness and honesty about eating and weight gain. We said to M at the beginning of FBT that we were going to treat her at home, that she was going to sleep in her own bed and that there was going to be no more facilities and no more programs. Also, we said that she was going to see an FBT therapist once a week whose function was to guide us through mandatory refeeding. There would be no arguments, no alternatives. M would also know what her target weight would be to be "refed," and every week she would see her progress toward that weight. The goal was to gain 1-2 pounds a week. Deal with it. In the early phases, she had no control, all decisions and meals were up to us. She stayed out of the grocery story during shopping, and she stayed out of the kitchen during meal prep. She would come into the kitchen when we told her, and she would eat whatever we had plated. We would also sit and eat the same food with her at the same time. She had one job, and that was to comply and eat and not hide food and to not vomit afterward.

I know this sounds crazy, but going straight at the heart of the demon, in the light of day, with your plan out in the open, is the best therapy. Like a championship football team, we broke the huddle, came up the line of scrimmage to get set, we pointed at the middle linebacker and said, "Our fullback is going to run this play right up your ass," and then we did it.

We made "treatment" and "therapy" actual actions instead of a process. There were no group discussions about feelings or coping skills. There was no one-on-one discussion about her fears and future goals. We decided to go full physiological to beat the psychological. Get her to the weight by bullying the state. Scare the fuck out of her demon by making her eat. Hell or high water. We metaphorically put her target weight up on a scoreboard and then said that she was going to eat like hell to get there. And we had no fear, we took time off work, we cancelled our social life, and we planned to ignore our family and friends for however long it took. We pushed the act and process of feeding M like a charging bull, on a strict schedule, and with the resolve of SEAL Team 6. She was going to eat until we said she didn't have to. We reset the fear parameters against the demon.

At the very beginning of M's slide into anorexia, body image was everything for her, and that was the genesis and the oracle of her weight loss. M's disordered thoughts started when she went through puberty at age 11, though we didn't know it at the time. She had one year where her body morphed itself completely. She went from shorter and wider, to suddenly taller and skinnier. Not in a bad way, but quite a growth spurt. Along with her body's growth spurt, she stopped her daily intake of noodles with butter and cheese and went to fruit and proteins and water. Nothing alarming at the time, and even her doctor saw the change and indicated that some kids can just hit a turning point. We have since learned that while M was not yet under the influence of the demon at that point, she was suddenly hyperaware of her body image and her calorie intake. These were new thoughts that she had never had before, so with no experience to learn from, and the fact she was only a young eleven-year-old, she started listening to these thoughts.

She would count calories and look at herself in the mirror every night. She would take dozens of pictures with her friends and then spend hours in her room comparing herself to them. And then there was the infinite and nauseating litany of Instagram posts by every girl in the world trying to look like a swimsuit model, and M added that content to her comparison drill. (Since these were curated and filtered versions what a woman "should look like," of course M would never measure up.) The point here is M's eating disorder started psychologically and led to disordered behavior in order for her to achieve a physical image that was not real nor realistic nor healthy.

M has talked to us about her journey both before the time we discovered her disorder, and in the time since we have been treating it. She has shared how she saw and understood her body image and eating behaviors. M felt that her only sense of power or equity came from her looks. She never considered her intelligence, her athletic abilities, her sense of humor, or her intrinsic goodness. She only saw her figure and appearance as her coin of the realm. Eating less food made her feel powerful, because she could affect how she looked and that created happiness. But as she lost more weight, she physically became weaker, and the disorder became stronger. We all saw a deteriorating form and a hollowed-out soul, whereas she saw thinner legs and a wider thigh gap and smaller shoulders. She was becoming so intoxicated and under the control of the demon voice that reality didn't penetrate. She was sinking into the quicksand both mentally and physically, both state and weight.

Ours is one story of how this poisonous weed takes root and infects an entire ecosystem that is a child. The vines wrap around the brain, the sense of reality, the clear outlook, the instinctive natural urges, and then the ability to see evil and take corrective action. This is about how mental illness kept a young woman out of school and teenage life and lead to self-harming behaviors. This is about how an eating disorder, specifically anorexia, is a mental disorder. And it is NOT just a girl problem, as boys are just as susceptible to the demon but are drastically under-diagnosed. This is serious shit that can affect any human being who has a brain and who eats.

As with all mental disorders and illnesses, there is an instinct by anyone involved or connected to run for the hills. Hide it, rename it, redirect attention. I have one friend in her twenties who described her teenage eating disorder like this. "I was first hospitalized and diagnosed over 10 years ago. At that time, patients in the facility I was in had a common cover story of having a 'heart issue,' which while technically true for myself, did not address the reason why I was having said cardiac issues."

I will write elsewhere in this book about the alarming number of eating disorders I do not see in everyday life. But when I poke my head into Dr. Knight's office, or into Stanford Hospital's eating disorder clinic, the vast prevalence of them in our society is overwhelming. It's like a character in an alien horror movie who puts on the secret glasses and sees how big the alien invasion really is, how all the aliens have hidden themselves in human form.

"Secrecy and control are everything," said a friend who I used to work with. Just before I left the wine industry to care for M full time, I was tasting wine with this friend when M called me. I excused myself to chat with M, but didn't leave the table. Whatever it was that I said to M on the phone, obviously something about eating, triggered a reaction in this friend. When I hung up, she politely asked who that was and was everything alright. I was very honest about treating M's anorexia via FBT, and that caused her to turn white with shock. She opened up about having been bulimic from age 14-28, that her parents never knew, and that she had only in the past few years really sought the counseling and treatment she needed to stop. She immediately went from "customer" to "confidant." Over the past three years, I have often sought her perspective and guidance, and sometimes just reached out to her to cry.

Her simple declaration about secrecy and control is germane to two sets of people. First and foremost, it is important to the kid who suffers from an eating disorder, because the demon demands that you lie and hide and manipulate so that no one treats that kid and the demon will prosper. Secondly, it applies to the people who surround that kid. Secrecy and control are the foundation for so much of the problem I am getting at here. I do not have the answer or explanation for peoples' lack of honesty about having an eating disorder, because I cannot find them to ask them. The patients and the families are all keeping it a secret and controlling what people know.

But for all the kids and young adults who have eating disorders and are not getting help, they need to start by asking themselves some simple questions or admitting some basic truths. Do you avoid eating, repeatedly? Do you overeat and then throw up? Do you take bites that you then spit up? Are you obsessed with all elements of your body's appearance to the point that it creates anxiety about eating? And maybe you know all this and have sought help. If so, have you been honest and open with your family and friends about your condition or that you may need more help? Are you seeing a doctor who specializes in eating disorders? Have you reached out to a therapist or psychologist who specializes in eating disorders? Have you been to the National Eating Disorders Association website (https://www.nationaleatingdisorders.org) to look for resources near you?

Yeah, this is all very rhetorical, but my point is that most likely the answer to everything in the previous paragraph is a big, fat "NO." Or the answer is a big, fat "I don't want to talk about this, I don't understand my feelings, I'm not going to be some weird, skinny supermodel sicko, lots of my friends act this way, my parents don't think I'm sick, I'm too scared to talk to my parents, I look great in my clothes, I finally made the dance team, OMG I love her Instagram." All of these hallmarks of denial can be found in most mental disorders, so I am not turning over any new soil, here. What I am pointing out is that all the denial issues surrounding the normal alcoholism and drug addiction, the ones we are more familiar with, need to be accepted as blocking people from eating. We all need to see that eating disorders need the same interventions we perform on the drunk and drugged. Eating while anorexic is just like driving while under the influence. There is no clear thinking or rational decision-making. Harm and death for at least one person is inevitable.

Chapter 3

The Richard Doctrine

Early in M's treatment for anorexia, she lived in a residential care facility for two months with five other kids, locked up in a big house on a secluded property with a full-time staff. M was forced to sit side-by-side with these other kids all day either eating or listening to therapy. She was watched like a hawk by the staff when she ate, went to the bathroom, showered, or sat on the porch. And the worst part was that she was forced to eat a lot of food. She wasn't happy in the slightest bit.

The Director and head therapist for this facility, Richard, would work with M a few times a week. This would entail a couple of one-on-one therapy sessions with M to discuss food fears and body image, and then there was our one family session for about 90 minutes to see how we could all support M's recovery. Richard was very bright and an accomplished professional in the eating disorder treatment community. He was one of the first to walk Tina and me through the dark corners and side roads of anorexia. He had worked with hundreds of kids and was very honest and direct with all of us.

The funniest and most poignant moment of M's time with Richard living in residential treatment (what we simply call "rez") and all of our time counseling with him and talking to him offline, came about midway through M's stay. We were having a family session, which back then was just M crying and arguing about anything any of us said. M started screaming that she did not have any problems with food, that she was just fine, and that she needed to be let out of this place right away. She continued by saying that Richard was stupid and that all the food sucked and that all this therapy was a waste of time. She concluded her rant by asking what the fuck all this was about? What the hell did we all want from her? Richard took off his glasses, rubbed his eyes, sighed and said, "M, you just gotta fucking eat."

I hope you can see the beauty of this, coming from this heavily educated and highly employed treatment professional, as he sits in the facility where he is the Director. For all the medical implications, the psychological and psychiatric necessities, and for all of the years of destruction to one's body and soul that comes from having an eating disorder, the basic answer and roadmap to freedom and recovery is simply that—you just gotta fucking eat.

If you ignore the rest of this book and learn nothing else about eating disorders, know this: the only cure to an eating disorder, specifically anorexia, is to keep eating until your body is strong and until you make peace with food. You keep eating until eating isn't an issue anymore, and your biggest stress is a bad hair day. A human being has to eat to survive and cannot go through life having a bad relationship with food. Consider other disorders, and the consequences of struggling or failing to break up with them: you can actually live for years as a functioning alcoholic or druggie or gambler. But you cannot physically survive short term or long term without food, not to mention that probably eighty plus percent of socializing with other people is done around food. Cooking food is the basis for romances and family holidays and television shows. Going to the market, or the farmers' market, is fun because you get to discover new foods and flavors. Traveling the world, or making new friends of different nationalities or ethnicities, is great because you'll get exposed to new and interesting food.

If you live every day in fear of the next meal, or if you wonder if you can get away with skipping lunch, or if you think you should blow off that date or friend meeting because you don't want to eat… that's no way to live. You just gotta fucking eat.

We declared those words to be "The Richard Doctrine," and we reference them often. But I use that as the chapter title and tell that story in order to highlight the big question: how do I get my eating disorder patient to just fucking eat? How do we beat the demon, and turn the war-ravaged mind of a child with an eating disorder into a peaceful place? How do I treat and beat this thing?

In the big picture, and remember this is my interpretation, there are initially two choices of how to get treatment: go away or do it at home with help. Either use an institution or stay in-house. Here is what I mean by this distinction. Once you no longer need hospitalization to keep the patient alive and he / she is stable, the refeeding has to start immediately. You have to tackle the "weight" issue until such a time as the patient is recovered physically to the point of being able to accept psychological therapy to address the "state" of mind issues. Are you as a person, as a married couple, as relatives or foster parents strong enough to take this on at home through Family Based Treatment (FBT), or do you need to send the patient away to live in a residential program or go to a daily outpatient facility?

Let's start with sending the patient, your child, away from home. In the very beginning, we had just learned that not only did M have a mental disorder, but it was the disorder with the highest mortality rate, and that M could have easily died if we had not gotten her into the hospital. We were a wreck, but there's no rest break in this process. We tried initially to do FBT when M came out of the hospital the first time, but we did not have the tools nor the information and experience we needed, and we got nowhere with her refeeding. We were referred to a company that runs many residential treatment facilities across the country, because it was clear that M needed "a much higher level of care." We got caught up in believing that getting M into a full-time program would be so much better for her. And I will completely admit, I love to hire subject matter experts to handle tasks that confound me: house painting, auto repair, tax preparation, you name it. And here was an opportunity to get rid of the demon that scared me so much and let someone else deal with it.

We gave M the heads up on a Friday night in late August 2019 that she was going to be admitted to a local residential facility on the following Monday. She had only been out of the hospital for three weeks and had only gone back to school for the first two weeks of her sophomore year. Tensions and anger and shit storms were high around our house, so we truly felt like this was our best move. We thought we knew how to handle FBT, but as I will address later, we did not. Tina and I were interviewed for about 90 minutes on the phone by the residential treatment facility company covering everything you could imagine about M's health, our family dynamic, her social tendencies, suicidal history and self-harming. Plus, Dr. Knight, the one who initially got her into the hospital, was the attending ED physician for this particular facility, so her referral bolstered our application.

What really surprised me at the time was that getting admitted to this residential treatment facility ultimately came down to whether or not we could afford it. The company that owns the facility had a whole process for getting insurance approval for admissions before even interviewing us. This place cost $1200 per day, and they wanted to know that payment would be forthcoming. As a matter of fact, one of Richard's jobs was to talk weekly to the insurance company of each patient to share progress reports and justify how much more time was needed to stay there. Insurance companies would then approve another 6-10 days at a time before needing to be convinced again.

In the week before we admitted M to the facility, we were getting more than one person saying that M needed a higher level of care, so I asked a different therapist how long M would need to stay there. How long does it take to cure this disorder? The therapist told me that as soon as the insurance company stops paying, the treatment is over and you better hope your kid is close to being cured.

The residential facility was near to where we lived and was a big house with a second outbuilding on about two acres. There were beds for six kids across three bedrooms, there were offices and treatment rooms, a huge kitchen and great room, outside gardens and a big wrap-around porch. It was a lovely setting, but it was still a restricted building. We had to be signed in and out every time we visited. On the morning of her intake, we were all unsure of what lay ahead, but M was a zombie. Knowing that she was going into this place that Monday, she later told us she had stopped eating food over that prior weekend. She figured, fuck it, I'm going away. Might as well abide by my demon if they are going to start trying to kill it on Monday.

When we got there, they took all her bags and belongings to search them and return anything not allowed. Things that could be used as weapons were not allowed, no makeup was allowed, and shorts were not allowed because patients cannot look at each other's legs to compare skinniness. Also, no phones or computers were allowed. No internet, no texting, no Snapchat, no Instagram. All contact with the outside world was in writing, or over the landline phone in the kitchen with a facility employee listening.

The best way to describe M's treatment in rez is formulaic and sterile. M was not allowed to get off the couch and walk until she fully complied with eating a certain number of meals. If she refused or restricted eating, she had to supplement the uneaten calories by drinking a supplement. Her bathroom breaks were monitored, and she couldn't flush until the toilet bowl was inspected. They watched her, indirectly, when she showered. All of this control was, somewhat rightly so, in pursuit of eliminating all disordered behavior around eating food, hiding food, and vomiting up food. But this environment overwhelmed M and brought on increased levels of anxiety and fear. Her demon thrived and shut down her ability to eat or relate to therapy. M was ultimately intubated with a nasogastric tube, NG for short. The tube allowed liquid supplement to be sent up her nose and down her throat into her stomach at mealtime. That was her way of eating for a couple of weeks.

At some point, you have to come home and live your life and take care of yourself. All the forced feeding and restrictions can have so many unintended side effects that derail true recovery. M tells us that rez was often a group of convicts sharing tips for fighting back against the institution: hiding food and rigging their weigh-ins. M also knew that while everyone who worked there was very committed and caring, it was still just where they worked. If M was not a successful patient or insurance stopped paying, another kid would take her place and M would soon be forgotten. The whole formula of rez is a good model for hope and for business, but it is really only a stopping over point on a years' long journey. You will often hear, see, and read about kids who do multiple stints in rez, similar to other recovery stories of alcohol and drugs. Kids who are struggling and recover just enough to get discharged and go back out on their own to often fail.

The step down from rez is outpatient treatment in the form of full-day or half-day therapy, depending on the needs, living situation or, again, insurance coverage of each patient. PHP refers to "partial hospitalization program," which M was placed in Monday through Saturday from 11:00AM to 7:00PM. IOP was the same outpatient program, but for folks who only needed a few hours a day after school. These facilities have therapists, dieticians, psychologists, and psychiatrists, all who work with the kids individually, in group settings, and with families. The kids learn to feed themselves by eating several of their meals and snacks there each day. And as much as I was blown away by the quality of the treatment professionals who worked there, it was still where they worked. There is a reasonable amount of latitude these folks should get from parents, as they must lose and gain patients all the time and move forward. If a kid washes out of there or has bad insurance, they have other kids to work with.

The final distinction for me about institutional treatment versus FBT, at least for the places where M was treated, is that some institutions believe in turning over meal planning to the patient way too early on in the recovery process. They believe that patient ownership of food is key. And while it generally is a good goal to get an ED patient in charge of their own meal plan and prep, I think their plan puts too much of key treatment in the hands of someone with no strength to handle it. Early in treatment when refeeding is key to basic health and sobriety, kids are too much under the control of the demon and cannot make the correct decisions that will lead to recovery. When M would put together one of her meals during PHP, she would prepare insufficient meals for her recovery plan, and then argue with us that these foods and portions had already been blessed by the program she attended.

One subset of this treatment philosophy, used at her rez and PHP, is referred to as "exchanges." There is an entire book about "exchanges" devoted to assigning points to every portion that is consumed of different kinds of food. Once memorized (as most OCD-minded eating disorder patients are prone to do) all these disordered kids will swear allegiance to this system and remain rigid in their acceptance of it for preparing meals. (Remember, meals are medicine. Meals are the cure. Meals need to outweigh the sickness). The goal of a meal built with exchanges is to target a daily total value of points across six categories: starch, protein, vegetables, fruit, dairy, and fat.

On September 29th of 2019, for example, M's worksheet for the day said she needed 13, 12, 2, 3, 4, & 12 points, respectively. So then for each of her six meals (three big ones, three snacks) a specific measurement of each component was listed and then its categorical value was checked off. At breakfast, 2/3 cup of vanilla Greek yogurt was 2 proteins. At lunch, 2/3 cup corn and 2 tbsp Italian dressing was 1 starch and 2 fats. Just skimming through the book itself, I read in the category "Starches," ½ cup pasta equals ½ cup white rice and counts as "1 starch." Under "Proteins," 2 slices of bacon equals 1 ounce of dried salami or 1 egg and counts as "1 protein and 1 fat." This is such a messed-up way of enslaving the mind of someone who loathes food and obsesses over quantities. Getting these kids so handcuffed to a rigid system, that as of now that I write this book has been discontinued and disavowed by that company, will create a huge roadblock long-term when they need to have an open relationship with any and all foods. Eating by formula is just another disordered way of eating.

Let's now look at bringing the care of your child in-house, no more facilities, no more employees and no more exchanges. I've already told the story of M putting herself back into the hospital a second time to get stabilized, right before Thanksgiving 2019. When that week was over, Tina and I brought M home and went to work with FBT. This is the scariest form of treatment, it affects everyone who lives at home, it somewhat isolates and insulates you from the outside world, but in the words of the greatest psychologist that we have ever met, it is the gold standard.

The first time Tina and I tried FBT, after M's initial hospital stay, we didn't have the right tools to be successful. And by the right tools, I mean we didn't have an FBT therapist. During M's second hospital stay, we were sitting with the hospital's in-house psychiatrist, and she asked us about our discharge plan. When we said we were going to try FBT, again, she then asked who our FBT therapist was. It was kind of like a "who's on first?" moment. We talked about having a therapist for M, but this woman quickly saw that we didn't know what we didn't know. We never knew that we needed a specific FBT therapist. These folks are fewer and further between, but they are the key to this whole thing. Tina and I thought that M needed just a therapist to talk to who knew about ED, which was fine, but an FBT therapist works with the whole family. Actually, the FBT therapist wants to work with the parents just as much or more and acts like a referee or mediator. And she sets and helps families maintain the rules.

We met Dr. Vandana Aspen a few years before when M first showed signs of a wicked case of OCD. As an accomplished athlete, M spent a lot of time on turf fields. At some point, M started to obsess about the dangers of chemicals, and then she projected all that fear onto artificial turf and how she believed it was going to kill her. Dr. Aspen specialized in working with OCD kids and believed in exposure therapy. By the time M and Dr. Aspen had spent four months of weekly therapy sessions together, M had rolled around in turf, put turf in her bed, and had walked through our house with her turf-stained cleats on. And guess what? She lived. It all cleaned up and went away, and M went on to become an even more accomplished athlete who played on turf. Face the fear. The only way out of or around something is through it. Dr. Aspen beat M's first demon.

So, when we came out of the hospital the second time with anorexia, committed to no more institutions, committed to beating this thing at home, we started looking for a therapist who specialized in FBT with anorexic kids. Guess who came highly recommended? Yup, Dr. Aspen. And man, what a difference she made.

FBT is for parents who are willing to say "no" to their kids. FBT is for parents who are not afraid to be a parent. FBT is another kind of exposure therapy, and in our first meeting, Dr. Aspen looked at all of us and laid down the rules. "M, not eating is not an option. You are in quicksand and your parents are here to pull you out. If you don't eat, you will die. You will eat whatever they plate for you, you will not hide food, and you are going to gain weight until we hit a target that a medical doctor determines is safe and healthy for you." And that, my friends, is the gold standard. Honest and direct, everyone on the same page, treatment at home by loving relatives who are not afraid of you and who are on duty 24/7/365.

Our weekly meetings with Dr. Aspen had great ups, but horrible downs. For example, unlike most other institutional approaches that don't show anorexia patients their weight, FBT is about exposure. You have to know your weight, it's just a number, plus it's a major metric in recovery. Staying blind to it is counterintuitive. So, every appointment started with M going into Dr. Aspen's office without us to catch up on the previous week, vent any issues in private, and finally get M's weight. Tina and I would then come in for the rest of the hour. Dr. Aspen set a simple recovery goal of 1-2 pounds a week of gain until M hit her target weight. Early on, M was averaging 3 pounds of gain per week, and it would set her off. She hated the weight gain, she screamed at us for going too fast and forcing too much food. She swore she was going to call Dr. Knight and tell her that the *&$&#@$ target weight was too high. Those drives home afterward were torture.

The good part about these weekly meetings was they ultimately culminated in M getting used to seeing her weight and hearing our concerns in a neutral setting. We could strategize new foods for the week or changes in portions. It felt like whatever was discussed in those meetings, and then was validated or blessed by Dr. Aspen, became the rules for the next week. And M generally stuck to these rules.

The six days in between our weekly sessions became somewhat rhythmic. M would generally eat all the meals we put in front of her, though early on she negotiated for no midmorning snack by agreeing to a bigger breakfast and bigger lunch. And while Tina and I oversaw all shopping, cooking and plating, allowing M to have some influence on meal choices or ingredients gave her some relief from her anxiety. It gave her a small sense of control. Our initial couple of months of FBT were all about "weight" and making sure she ate to get back to a physically sober status. M tried to argue for exchanges, but we refused and told her to let go of that thinking. And while Dr. Aspen told Tina and me to not focus too much on calories, that was all we secretly did. As I point out in other parts of this book, calories became our greatest weapon, and it put the pounds back on quickly. At one point when M was angry about our food and that she was gaining too much weight too fast, Dr. Aspen put it to her simply. "M, the faster we go, the less time you have to wallow in this. Let's rip off the band-aid and get there sooner." M didn't acknowledge the wisdom in this at the time, but she still kept eating whatever we served her.

Another thing Tina and I didn't have the first time we tried FBT was experience and information. And one example those are the books about the Maudsley approach, especially those written by Eva Musby There are so many memoirs and overviews of life with eating disorders that you can read, but by reading and starting with Eva's books, which are specifically about FBT, you will find great help. You will see and hear that you are not alone, and that every fight and episode you go through at home is standard operating procedure for this process. Eva's books lays out scripts for you to follow when dealing with the demon, and they also show you how effective empathy can be. You will also see how this road to recovery is ultimately the best. You must be willing to stand up not only to your kid, but actually up to their demon and for your kid, and you have to be willing to be the bad guy. Be the parent. There are legions of writings out there by older and recovering eating disorder patients who say that they cannot remember all the specific fights and terrible words yelled, but they remember being grateful and comforted knowing their parents were fighting for them when they could not fight for themselves.

We are now years into FBT. And while we still have struggles with the demon and rigid thinking, those struggles are further up Maslow's Hierarchy of "Problems." And we couldn't have gotten here without committing to FBT and sticking to our guns. At this point, M just fuckin' eats.

Chapter 4
The Information Gap

I have nothing but the highest and utmost respect for anyone in the medical field. Doctors, Nurses, Counselors, you name it. If you have studied and trained, and then committed your life to improving the health and well-being of others, you are a way better person than me. And when I am in need, I'm coming to you for help.

What I mean to discuss in this chapter is where I may get into trouble, but it's what I have seen firsthand. There is a rampant lack of education and information for health professionals about eating disorders, and it parallels a similar track in the private sector.

When I was first spiraling into the fear about M's weight issues in the early summer of 2019, we saw M's skeleton every day under her bikini. Tina and I decided to make a doctor's appointment for M under the guise of getting her cleared for fall sports in high school. We called her normal pediatrician ahead of time and laid out our concern for M's health vis-a-vis her weight and eating issues. When we got to the appointment, M went in to see the pediatrician on her own first. After a while, Tina was asked to go in. This was the first time anyone with authority (the pediatrician) had confronted M about her weight loss, and it caused M to break down in tears. The pediatrician went so far as to play the "bad guy" and said she would not sign M's clearance for fall sports in high school until she got her weight back up. The pediatrician also referred us to a dietician to work with M. YES! We have figured this out and we have a plan to fix this.

No.

No, we did not.

We were delusional, and this pediatrician had barely done us a favor.

Based on several conversations that I have since had with practicing physicians of various ages, they have all told me that they experienced a very minimal amount of instruction about eating disorders in medical school. Most of the folks I spoke to described their length of training using the phrase "part of a day, maybe." I keep this in perspective by imagining the infinite litany of biology, chemistry, physiology, anatomy and probably alchemy that must be bestowed upon would-be doctors. The information in medical school is beyond vast, and by the time any of these folks get around to continuously working with patients, they have started to specialize in various fields so as to focus their skills and knowledge base. No one can know everything.

However, the fact remains that most physicians and hospitals are not currently set up to diagnose and treat eating disorders. One group of veteran emergency room physicians that I spoke to said that, though they understand the connection between low heart rates and orthostatia and even dehydration in a patient who is suffering from the demon, they would not immediately initiate "treat eating disorder" protocol. If anything, they would mostly likely just address the short-term issues in order to physically and medically stabilize the patient. They also told me that, unlike many other situations where they might come across symptoms that they are not familiar with and thus call a specialist, none of these folks knew of a reliable eating disorder expert to consult. Doctors are "fixers," meaning they love to and want to treat or cure or medicate or set or bandage or fix. It is hard to put a leash around an eating disorder and lead it to a fix.

Even beyond the immediate treatment of a patient presenting physical symptoms of eating disorders, a lot of physicians see eating disorders as being owned by the realm of psychology, and that those psychologists will manage these patients and know when to initiate medical help. The physicians also felt that the knowledge and awareness of eating disorders was pervasive enough, but the shortfall in the medical community was the lack of resources to treat it. Eating disorders are, after all, looked upon as mental disorders right up there with depression, suicide, and bi-polar disorder, all of which have treatment protocols that are very underfunded.

On the brighter side, one younger physician I spoke with introduced me to a field of study and focus that has gotten more attention over the last eight to ten years called "The Female Triad." This initially concentrated on young women who were physically active, usually competitive athletes, and how this affected three parts of their bodies: disordered eating, amenorrhea, and osteoporosis. We all know about disordered eating, which can range from light malnutrition to full-on anorexia or bulimia. But when you see that mixed with decreased hormones and thus irregular or flat out missing menstrual cycles (amenorrhea), and then also mixed with the weakening of bone density and development (osteoporosis), a bigger and more horrific picture develops.

I say "brighter side" because now physicians were sweeping together a lot of the smaller signs of how a raging mental disorder presents itself physically in a patient and naming a diagnosis for it. And this was leading physicians to address the whole disorder instead of hoping that a psychologist could help. To highlight how much attention this field of study was getting, "The Female Triad" was recently renamed "Red-S" to stand for "Relative Energy Deficiency in Sports." This new name takes the approach that all of these ailments can also happen in men, as well, minus the amenorrhea. And now some of the specific diagnosable signs of Red-S are also very specific to anyone, athlete or not, who has an eating disorder: fatigue, hair loss, (yet, ironically, increased body hair growth to keep the thinner structure warm), cold hands and feet, dry skin, noticeable weight loss, increased healing time from injuries (e.g., lingering bruises), increased incidence of bone fracture, low self-esteem, and depression. This means that eating disorder symptoms are becoming a common focus within family medicine and pediatrics, but again, it is a newer field, and it still has not had its fifteen minutes of fame.

It is important to note that eating disorders were not always classified as mental illnesses by the American Psychiatric Association. Their book, *Diagnostic and Statistical Manual of Mental Disorders* (DSM), is the commonly accepted benchmark that determines whether a mental condition is considered a medical issue. Anorexia has long been accepted as a medical issue and was identified in the first edition of the DSM in 1952. Yet bulimia was not added to the DSM until 1987, and binge-eating, and Avoidant Restrictive Food Intake Disorder (ARFID) were not separately identified until 2013. Once each of these are identified in the DSM, then insurance companies will consider offering coverage for treatment, but not always.

Going back to the first pediatrician appointment, I do not have the actual vitals as measured on that day, but M's pediatrician had an eleven-year history of her BMI, her height, and her weight all on file and on the chart in front of her. While the value of each data point may not be the whole story, the trend over time should have sounded the alarm bells. M, on that day, was 24 days away from being admitted to the hospital. This pediatrician, while doing her best, either did not see or was not trained to see the declines and the signs. The dip in M's BMI and growth curve were scary, her lack of a menstrual cycle for a long time was telling, and the visually apparent weakness in her frame was glaring. Yet, no warning was sounded. In fact she said "M will be just fine."

It took us ten more days to get into the dietician, who was really impressive. As much as Tina and I thought we knew about food, this was a whole new way to examine intake and variety and volumes. We were so impressed with how she worked with M that Tina and I each signed up to evaluate our own eating plans. Again, this is all great information, but it was no match for the demon that was consuming M. We were given an eating plan for M in the form of a picture of a dinner plate that showed the percentages of carbs, fats, proteins, and vegetables that M should eat at each meal. This was not going to address the deeper self-image problems, nor the eating restriction issues M was having. It was just another method to stoke a fight with M when we tried to feed her.

I spend a lot of this book telling you to educate yourself about the sources of disordered thinking around food, as well as my opinion about how best to treat the disorder. What I mean to bring up in this chapter is that just because you go to a doctor or dietician, don't think that you have the problem, or the treatment, covered. They know how to help kids with the flu and broken ankles and UTIs, or with sports training and recovery eating. They do not all know how to identify, diagnose, and treat eating disorders. I have joked that eating disorders have not yet gotten their 15 minutes of fame along the lines of, say, breast cancer. When the NFL has a "Breast Cancer Awareness" week where all the players wear pink and they raise millions of dollars and awareness, you have to figure that the medical community is ready to give the best possible treatment to anyone diagnosed with breast cancer. Eating disorders, not so much.

There is also a huge issue with parents. They may

not take their kid's weight loss that seriously, and if they do, they blow it off as teenage obsession with appearance or praise an overweight child because this is bringing their weight down. They may just figure that their kid is trying to eat healthy. Or, in a worst case scenario, they don't notice at all. And even if they do notice, and get their kid diagnosed, and get sucked down the hole to the hell, they don't acknowledge it or talk about it. They feel ashamed or want to give their kids privacy. They whitewash it.

When M was diagnosed and went fully off the rails early on, her best friend was right there by her side. (Thanks, E!) And her friend's dad, a longtime soccer sideline buddy of mine, was right there, too. (Thanks, Tom) He checked in on me almost every day. And the most telling conversation I have ever had about eating disorders, I had with him. He and I had each been in our community for 12-15 years. We had been a part of dozens of soccer and lacrosse leagues, school groups, clubs, you name it. Between the two of us, we touched hundreds of local families. You want to know how many instances of eating disorders we had ever heard of? One. M. No one else.

Total bullshit.

The mental disorder with the highest death rate ever diagnosed, prominent in high achieving communities, rampant and growing in an era of social media conflagration, and between the two of us we had never heard of it. No one had anything to contribute. Statistically, this was unheard of.

Eating disorders still live in the shadows because of the fear of the unknown, because of the lack of information, and because of the shame supposedly implied by the few facts and instances that are public and known. There needs to be a big "loud and proud" moment so that better information is readily available, and shame is no longer an issue. We cannot let the wrongly assumed stigma around a "skinny girl" disease keep a family from recognizing early on the signs that a child is struggling with food. Because that struggle can and will lead to years of mental terror, physical torture and possibly death. The earlier you intervene and start intense treatment, the quicker you will dispatch the demon. You will have a better chance of getting your kid clear of this disorder if you do not let it linger unattended. Once those rigid and blinding thoughts take root in your child and grow unchecked, the harder it will be to break your child free of those behaviors.

M went into the hospital for the first time in late July of 2019, and as I write this now, that memory brings tears to my eyes. That admission was five days after we took her to the initial pediatrician for a second visit about her weight. And though the pediatrician stuck to her guns about M not being fit enough to play high school sports, she put her arm around me and said, "M is going to be just fine." At one point during M's hospital stay, not out of spite but out of the spirit of communication, I called that same pediatrician to let her know that M had been admitted to the hospital for anorexia. The conversation was brief and quiet.

A couple of months later, one night when M was in rez and I was getting ready to head over for visiting hours, my phone rang from a local number. It was the pediatrician. It was well after hours and she was very careful and measured in her speech. She asked how M was doing. When I laid out the hospital visit, the failed FBT treatment, and now the residential stay, the pediatrician said she had recently seen a lot more patients presenting symptoms of anorexia and that she was working more closely with the company that ran M's facility.

I have absolutely no bad feelings toward this pediatrician, and I only tell this story because I think that M's situation became a wakeup call that this doctor didn't know was coming. Eating disorders are not a part of the daily language that a lot of physicians speak. There hasn't been the fifteen minutes of fame, yet. Families are not recognizing the symptoms and signs, nor are they asking the medical community for help. Education, information, admission, and acceptance will go a long way to making eating disorders easier to deal with, both medically and emotionally.

Chapter 5
Fuck You Eggs

The first thing I ever learned to cook was eggs. It was somewhere in the mid 1970s, and it was omelets to be specific. My parents had an omelet pan, I guess that's what it was called, and it was called that for the following reason. It's a round pan, very deep (high sides), but it is hinged in the middle. So, looking down from left to right, you have a round pan broken into two half-moons. You pour part of your whisked eggs into each side, cook them until ready, and then grab the handle that was on one of the sides, and you flipped it over. Perfect half circle omelet. I remember putting in some cheese, but not much else.

Also, around that time in my life, I had a pediatrician named Ed Bronski. He was a really nice man—my folks even became friends with Ed and his wife. He was originally from New York but moved out to Salt Lake City for medical school and never left. When I got sick, my mother would always make me a runny egg on toast and say that Dr. Ed prescribed it to make me feel better. It was called an "Ed Special." To this day, my son knows that story and will refer to that dish by name as he cooks it for himself.

At this point in life, I'm a pretty good cook, and I've always been really into reading cookbooks, watching cooking shows and demos, and constantly tinkering with recipes. I love feeding my family and friends and being the person making a mess with lots of tasty food to eat. I have three barbecues—getting up at 5:00 in the morning to start the fire to smoke brisket while drinking espresso (thanks, Aaron) makes me happy. I was even given a chef's jacket by my family, with the moniker "Fat Camp Executive Chef" embroidered into it because long family weekends of eating at our house are called "Fat Camp." You get the picture.

Tina is also a great cook, so we spend a lot of time in the kitchen together as a family. And while our primary mantra to our kids has always been, "solve the problem," a close second is "learn to feed yourself." Our kids know how to make Christmas cookies and pumpkin bread, grilled sandwiches and BBQ, Italian and Mexican and Thai food. We live in the kitchen. The fucking fact that the disorder my daughter suffers from is a fear of food is insultingly ironic.

Like, *what*?

I have titled this chapter as such and told you stupid stories because there is a dish I make my recovering daughter that has taken on a weird status. We are right now at a point in her recovery where she is pouring all her own drinks, plating a few items throughout the day, and even pretty much making her own breakfast... though with lots of supervision and prep work by us. The point is, the one meal that M loves the most, the one meal that M jokingly tries to estimate the makings of, is a plate of scrambled eggs. She just calls them "eggs." I call them "fuck you eggs." Why? Follow along.

Every time you see a high-ranking official from the intelligence community testifying in front of a Congressional committee, at some point he / she is asked about the torture and waterboarding of terrorists, and what is their response? "Of course, we don't do that. We are able to root out and fight our enemy without resorting to those tactics. Those tactics are illegal."

Once I came to know that the demon of anorexia was a terrorist, who would stop at nothing to kill my daughter, who would know nothing of compromise or diplomacy, I then knew no amount of fighting dirty was off the table. And I was not about to negotiate with a terrorist. Over the long term of bringing your child out of an eating disorder, you cannot hide certain ingredients or foods, but in the beginning, it's all guns on deck. Initially, weight restoration is the key to getting your kid sober, bringing him or her back online with all systems: clear thinking, immune system, digestion and gastrointestinal, reproductive (no period for a year?), endocrine system, etc. You would bury your kid in a silo to keep them away from drugs or alcohol to get them back to sober, right? The goal of refeeding, of getting your kid to weight restoration, though just the first of many steps, is the same thing.

We resorted to some clandestine tactics to beat the demon-terrorist and this included concealment. For example, you have to hide calories in everything you make. You cannot simply plate some meal that looks like the lumberjack special at a diner. No, anorexia is that cyborg from Terminator whose vision of food has instant readouts and calculations about portion size, calories, fat, carbs, and proteins. It is even worse if your child has been to a residential facility or outpatient program that employs "exchanges" that boost disordered eating to another level.

Anyway, what you plate and present to your child during refeeding is an art and a science. First, consider what your family routines were before this disorder. Did you all eat lots of casseroles and pasta, usually just salads and smoothies, all meat or no meat, or drive-through fast food as a default? The past eating habits and food environment of your family will initially be a pattern that your child's disorder will measure against. Our family food outline was mostly made up of disparate elements of protein and vegetables and carbs, which any of us would combine to our individual wants. I'd roast chicken or grill skirt steak, smoke a pork shoulder or a brisket, and those leftover meats would always be in a refrigerator full of cheese, eggs, fruits, and vegetables. And that refrigerator was next to a pantry full of rice or pasta or tortillas. With Tina and I working full time, and both teenage kids busy, this base food always allowed someone to mix ingredients and prepare a meal for themselves. So, my challenge as someone who loves to cook, was to start with our old patterns, bury as much fat and calories into it, and move M forward into as much variety as possible.

When we first started FBT, M's range of food was limited, and she didn't want to eat different foods. I kept talking about eggs, she kept telling me to fuck myself. At some point she agreed, no doubt through some kind of brokered deal with Dr. Aspen, to having scrambled eggs. So, I looked at a lot of eggs to find the most potent ingredients. What I learned, through a lot of trial and error, and a lot of calorie counting, was to skip the white ones and go with the brown ones because their yolks are a darker color. (This will matter) Next, I bypassed the large or XL size, and went for the jumbo eggs. And usually, I found that organic eggs carried more calories. What I ended up with was two different organic brown egg brands where each egg is 90 calories.

Next step is to consider how an egg is comprised. The vast amount of fat, cholesterol and calories are in the yolk. So, my base recipe became two full eggs and an additional yolk. (All the while, saving the whites to make other stuff for Tina and me. Funny side note: M has either never noticed the Tupperware of egg whites in the fridge, or hasn't thought to ask why they are there.) I added to these organic heavy whipping cream. There are 60 calories per tablespoon here, so I poured in two. That now is about 250 calories from eggs, mostly fat and protein, plus 120 calories of pure cream fat. What else should we mix in? Here is the silver bullet, widely debated but never underestimated: Benecalorie. Benecal, for short. Thank you, Nestle Corporation. 1.5 ounces of liquid sunflower oil, providing 330 calories of pure fat. Shake the small container of it for a long time before you open and pour. If there is any solid putty-like stuff left in there, just scrape it into the egg mixture.

Now it is time to whisk like your kid's life depends on it. Rake your fork through the mixture off and on, then comb around the sides of the bowl. After about a minute, it starts to resemble something normal. And if you are starting to get stage fright about how this is going to look or how on Earth you are going to get away with this, just remember that the magical process of high heat will save you.

Without taking away from the chapter of this book entitled, "A Matter of Thyme," there is a lot in the presentation of food that can absolve your sins. Get out a small skillet, and on the counter next to it, put a can of PAM nonstick spray. Make sure to hit the pan with a big spray of this stuff, not only for nonstick quality, but the sound of this spray to the kid upstairs or in the other room indicates lots of ZERO calorie additions. But still throw in two tablespoons of butter to melt in with the PAM. And as long as that PAM is sitting there, and your kid will notice it, the power of suggestion and the existence of that can will dissuade their potential protest later.

So where are we? 250 egg calories, 120 heavy whipping cream calories, 330 Benecal calories, and 200 butter calories. That gives us a total of 900 mostly fat-based calories.

Once the butter melts with the PAM at a low heat, pour in the egg mixture, and make sure to rubber scrape it all in. Also, do not ever deviate from obfuscation protocol: make sure that the ingredients bowl is rinsed in the sink so no evidence of your base concoction is evident, and make sure your Benecal container is hidden somewhere. (The inside bottom of my golf bag did the trick). Then, dump a bunch of thyme into the eggs, or dried basil, or dried oregano, or chives. Again, misdirection. Grind pepper and sprinkle in garlic salt.

Trust me, kids being refed love salt, and it gives them something that is zero calories to think about. All this color and flavor in the final mixture will dampen the demon's questions about any nefarious additions.

M loves crispy bacon and well-done steak. I highly encourage you to move your child toward that preference during recovery. Because any food that is overcooked, or blackened, or slightly burned, in no way takes on the appearance of its original ingredients.

With the stove still on low heat, gently stir and flip the eggs around, but also let the mixture sit at times to soak all the fats together. For most of the time I have been making this, I ultimately would get the eggs to a point where I had browned all the bits, but it was fluffy. Lately, M has asked me to make them into a frittata, so I brown both sides really well. I make sure all the butter is burned in, and the dark orange color of the brown eggs helps to hide any evidence of the Benecal.

Finally, put a folded over paper towel on the plate. When the eggs are done, I put them on the towel and fold it gently around the eggs to dab off excess greasiness, and then serve with a gluten-free Trader Joe's cracker that is 130 calories. Add a big cup of cranberry juice or soy milk at about 150 calories, and boom. You now have 1100-1200 calories in what looks like just a slightly larger-size egg portion. When your child asks what's in it, how many eggs did you use (oddly, they forget to ask about dairy or Benecal), you look into your child's eyes and say two very fluffy and seasoned eggs. You do it with pride and you do it with ego.

Fuck you, demon.

There are and can be so many variations, but think

of the fat. Fat is key. Fat sticks around. It doesn't burn off easily. All the 50-year-olds like me know that fat is hard to get rid of. It would visibly and proportionally take so many carbs and sugars to get this many calories into a meal. Plus, the protein and fat both go toward muscle development that weighs more. Take my recipe, take my approach, take my twisted thinking, and see your child's eating disorder as a terrorist. Torture and waterboard that motherfucker, because you cannot negotiate for weight restoration with a terrorist.

Once you move forward in FBT beyond weight restoration, your child will start taking small steps. Pouring their own drink or plating certain pieces of food, with supervision, are good steps. Starting to prep one or two pieces of food, with supervision, will also happen. But the problem with the malicious egg recipe above is that, if M wants to make it on her own, she'll have to see that stuff that I hid in it. A few years from now, she may be able to laugh about it, but not now. That's the problem with hiding or manipulating food in FBT: the ultimate goal is to turn back over to the child the power and responsibility of feeding themselves. If you as the refeeder in charge are scoring runs and gaining pounds through sleight of hand, you have to have an exit plan.

Going forward, I need to make a plate of scrambled eggs without Benecal that tastes and looks similar. Once she is used to that, maybe then I back down from the heavy whipping cream to half and half. (All the while, mind you, making sure she does not lose weight and slip backwards). I need to get the egg recipe to a point where I say, "Yup, you got me. It's 3 full eggs plus a yolk and some half & half." Whatever reaction M gives to that sentence will be mild compared to her response to knowing the real recipe. I expect she would even shrug and accept it, though she may not eat it again. I am ultimately trying to keep her trust, not trigger her into resisting my food.

(*Note inserted much later) What ultimately happened was that we eliminated the FU eggs from her diet in the name of "variety" and "other food exposure." As I write this, those eggs have not been made in months. If we are to go back to them, I think I can just try the 3 – 3.5 eggs plus half and half. So, we lucked out in not having to either fess up to their contents or try to alter their condition. If you find that you've painted yourself into a corner with a secret dish during FBT, try just stopping for a while so you don't get caught.

Chapter 6
Last Call

There are so many times when the treatment or the journey of a person with an eating disorder include the words "being hospitalized." It is absolutely true, and mostly mandatory, that many people with eating disorders end up in the hospital, though it is ironically often the last step *before* the first treatment actually starts. Admission into a hospital is usually the result of rapid weight loss or inadequate nutrition that leads to the loss of healthy physiology that manifests in low blood pressure and heartrate, weakness, fainting, fatigue, depression, anxiety, and other alterations in organ systems that inhibit their ability to, well, live. A visit to a doctor, or a visit by paramedics, usually instigates the patient going into a regular hospital or, if lucky, a specialized eating disorder ward. Once there, if your physician is well-informed and fluent in eating disorders, you will learn that your weak and withering child is not just a bit burned out and tired. You will learn that you have entered hell and that an eating disorder is currently trying to kill your kid. Welcome, come on in, the water's not so nice.

Upon admittance to the hospital, your child will

immediately be hooked up to a heart monitor, which will stay on the entire time he or she is there. This is ground zero, because when the body is starved of nutrients and fuel, the heart is the key organ that will fail right before you start making funeral plans. The most basic metrics that determine your child's need for hospitalization are those of the heart: heart rate, blood pressure, and the orthostatic change of both.

A healthy teenager should have a resting heart rate of 60-100 beats per minute. If they drop into the 50s, that could be cause for concern, though kids who are very athletic can naturally have that slow of a rate. Any rate in the 40s should raise the alarm, any rate in the 30s can lead some doctors and nurses to start CPR. (M was admitted to the hospital for the first time with a resting heart rate of 41 and an overnight heart rate in the 30s.) The point here is, such a slow rate of heart beats shows a drastic lack of fuel in the system.

Blood pressure is also key. I'm not going to go into all the numbers on this one, but weak and low blood pressure usually goes hand in hand with a low heart rate: if the heart is slow in pumping blood as a result of being malnourished, then often the pressure throughout the body is low. And when these two readings are low together, your child's health is in danger.

The final variable is the determination of the change in a patient's resting heart rate when compared against the rate when that patient stands up. If that change is in excess of 20 beats per minute, they have orthostasis or are referred to as being orthostatic. For example, think of two healthy teenagers who are sitting on the couch for 30 minutes watching a movie. One of them hits the pause button and they both get up to refill their drinks. They go from sitting to standing to walking and moving in an instant. A healthy teenager's heart will increase 5-20 beats per minute to support the body's need for blood flow to facilitate this new motion, no problem. A starved and deprived eating disorder patient will see an increase in their heart rate of 20-60 beats. They are in such a weakened state that the act of standing puts up to two or three times the power request on their heart just to facilitate the body's movements. This will usually lead to light-headedness and, all too often, a fall or fainting. M's orthostasis measurement was +60 the first time she was admitted to the hospital.

It is important to note that the affected patient being put into the hospital may not believe they feel poorly. "Anosognosia" is a common feature in eating disorders where the patient lacks the awareness or acceptance of the fact that they have a medical condition. This hallmark symptom leads the patient to say they feel fine, and to explain away any other eating disorder symptoms as the result of random and common occurrences. This sense of denial in the patient is one of the reasons it can be so hard to treat eating disorders.

Another mental roadblock in the mind of a child with an eating disorder, one that is a fundamental reason they are in the hospital, and one that will also make treatment very hard, is "Body Dysmorphia." This is where the patient cannot stop thinking about one or more perceived defects or flaws in their appearance—a flaw that appears minor or cannot be seen by others. These patients are preoccupied with imagined physical defects of their own bodies, especially in light of how they compare themselves to other people. This perspective often triggers the actions and behaviors of food avoidance and restriction, that in turn creates the inadequate nutrition mentioned earlier. Similarly, these patients also often have a distorted way of viewing the food they see on their plate, and perceive the amount as larger than it actually is.

So your kid has a heart monitor connected to their chest for the entire time they are in the hospital. The next order of business is to see what numbers that monitor spits out as a measurement of the heart's status. If your kid's heart rate, blood pressure, and orthostasis are all in the red, then bed rest is the prize. As in, other than going to the bathroom, the kid cannot get up. He or she reads, watches TV, eats, chats, texts, and looks out the window all from the bed. This is to give the heart the best chance to have the least amount of demand on it while it receives an increased level of nutrition and fuel. It also prevents falls and injury, because the kid is so malnourished that he or she is in the hospital, so it's highly likely they might faint. Finally, any and all movement that could burn or compromise a single calorie needs to be eliminated. This kid is in a MASH unit right now, being put back together, and everything counts. Not to mention, since so many kids with an eating disorder do an obscene amount of exercise to lose weight, this grounding of activity in bed helps to curb that thinking in the short term.

After being stuck in bed for a few days and eating six times a day, your kid's body starts to respond. They are getting the first meaningful and consistent input of calories and nutrition that they have had in quite a while. They are also getting desperately needed hydration. They may be having their first bowel movement in weeks, which will kick start other systems in the body. If all this moves the needle on all those heart metrics in a positive direction, then they are allowed to move around outside their bed in a wheelchair. Believe me, they will be so happy to move around and see other people. This mobility will then offer them one of their first choices since being admitted: would you like to continue to eat in your room with the nurse and your parents, or would you like to join the other patients on the ward in the group room for food? You might think that seeing other kids would be a huge lure, but remember, anyone who is hospitalized for an eating disorder is in a dark, depressed place. Seeing other kids like them isn't exactly a big "wow, yeah" moment. Kids in this place, physically, mentally, and emotionally, seek isolation and want to hide who they are. Even if your kid joins in a group meal, no one talks, and everyone silently battles for who can be the most sick and who can restrict the most amount of food.

There will finally come a day when your kid's vital signs are strong enough that they are allowed to get out of bed, get out of the wheelchair and walk on their own, wheeling their heart monitor around on a pole with them. There's really not much real estate in the hospital where they can walk, but they will feel the very first inklings of working hard to earn a small freedom. They may use this freedom to merely sit in the window sill of their room or go out onto a patio or balcony to feel some fresh air. They, and you, have no basis for knowing that this type of restricted and managed movement will happen again and again down the road if the eating disorder puts your kid into a residential program or you come back to the hospital. Even in an FBT environment, parents must clamp down on and forbid most movement and exercise until the calories take hold and the weight starts to stick. This control over a kid's sense of freedom will cause a tremendous amount of conflict down the road, but it is an absolutely necessary tool in the process of getting an eating disorder patient sober and weight restored.

And now we need to talk about eating, because the hospital is the first place you start to piece together the concept of a meal plan and a calorie goal. You are told by the doctors and nurses and dieticians, based on their observations of your kid and the actual vitals, what the weight restoration goal is and how much food per day they are going to feed that kid. And this is not negotiable. Each meal is built around all the food groups that will ultimately add up with the other meals to hit the daily calorie goal. You as a parent need to start seeing that equation and knowing what it needs to add up to.

Initially, some kids struggle to get 1000 calories into their system in one day. Think of how small some stomachs can get or how fragile a GI tract can be after being starved for a long period of time. As an analogy, consider an old, used sponge at your kitchen sink. You know, shriveled and dry and hard as a rock. Now put that sponge under running water. Initially, the water just bounces off, runs right over and around. Nothing penetrates. Slowly, water absorbs, and the sponge starts to retain moisture and develop a smaller and weaker shell of its former shape. This is your kid's body and how it takes in food after a long period of starvation. In the extreme, consider what you have read or heard about prisoners of war who are finally released after years of captivity. They were forced into disordered eating and mass malnutrition, and their recovery took years.

Eventually, you will need to move the daily calorie target up, again based on the weight deficit your kid created and the healthy size their body needs to be. It is very common that you will need to get 4000-6000 calories per day into your kid for months just to get back to weight restoration. And as I have said, or will say, elsewhere in this book: this is the hardest thing imaginable for this child, to do that which they fear and hate the most just so that they can be strong enough to battle the demon that is haunting them.

As you learn refeeding in the hospital, you are also taught about "supplementing." This means that when your kid gets to the end of their rope in a meal, or to say, they hit the wall and cannot finish the solid food on the plate because of the raging terror of the demon inside, or their stomach is bursting… well, the calorie plan cannot be compromised. It is time to supplement the calories left on the plate with a liquid substitute. Usually Ensure or Boost is used, and a quarter to a full bottle will do the trick. This is torture for the kid in a couple of ways. First, it's a slap in the face to the idea that they determine when they are done. Nope, those calories are coming one way or another. And second, the flavor and texture of any of the liquid meal substitute drinks can become unpleasant after a while to a person trying to embrace real food.

One of the worst-case scenarios to learn about when hospitalized for eating disorder recovery is the nasogastric tube, or NG. If your child is so tortured by the demon that they cannot physically consume food by putting it in their mouths and bring those calories to the fight in their stomach, then another way in must be found. The NG is a rubber tube that is inserted through the nose and is then fished down through the esophagus and into the stomach. Once this is done, while the kid is awake, they do an x-ray just to make sure the tube didn't accidentally go off and get stuck in a side alley somewhere. Finally, they take the top end of the tube coming out of the nose, loop it over the kid's ear and clip it to their shirt collar. Seriously, it looks like some Secret Service Agent's earpiece. Then, when it's mealtime, they unclip the tube from the shirt, attach it to a pump full of supplement, and down into the stomach goes the liquid load of calories. Yup, that kid sits there, in front of the nurse, and feels liquid food flow through their nose and down into their guts to pool up and nourish them. M had this tube for two and a half weeks.

The other part of refeeding that you as a parent learn at the hospital is that no meal goes unsupervised. You have to sit with your child at every meal and multitask like an octopus. You must vigilantly watch that all food goes into the mouth and is swallowed. The food is not spit down the shirt, into a closed hand, onto the floor, into a water bottle, or stuck on the roof of the mouth. You must see that all food that is pushed around the plate and squashed with the fork is not jettisoned off into a waiting napkin or under the sheets, or even down the waist band of the pants. All the while, you are supposed to calm the terrorized kid and help ease the tension of the moment by talking, or reading a book out loud, or watching TV, or doing a puzzle. What you cannot do is talk about food or eating or being in the hospital or having an eating disorder. And when, not if, the kid has a demonic flash and lashes out about hating you and hating being in the hospital and hating eating, you cannot engage. You must calmly redirect and be supportive… without talking about eating food.

At the end of your stay in the hospital, your kid has not been treated for an eating disorder. Your kid has been pulled back from the brink of serious injury or death. Your kid's vitals have been stabilized and your kid is just strong and healthy enough to walk out the door. That kid leaves the hospital when they no longer require hospitalization. As a part of that exit process, a hospital that specialized in eating disorders will consult with you about your after-hospital plan and will help you put together the assets you may need. Are you going to treat your child at home via FBT, and if so, do you have a FBT therapist? Who is your kid's physician, and is that physician well-informed about eating disorders? Do you need a psychiatrist to either continue or initiate medicine (anxiety pills), and are you going to use a dietician? If you are going to immediately enroll your kid into a residential or out-patient program, have you been accepted and does your insurance cover it? All these questions and decisions are so overwhelming to research, consider and decide in a calm environment...they are exponentially worse after the five or ten days you just spent not sleeping and worrying to death about your child's life and safety. Not to mention, you just got started with an understanding of what the hell an eating disorder is, and since no one fucking talks about eating disorders in our society because of the shame and lack of education, you probably have no one to call and ask for help.

Many eating disorder patients' stories will likely include at least one, if not multiple, stays in the hospital. That, though, is not where the real treatment happens. But it is where the alarm bells are sounded and where the gripping fear sets in. And it can also be where a parent's or family's resolve to fight this demon takes hold.

Chapter 7
Riding & Writing

I don't have a bucket list, but writing a book has always been a huge goal of mine. Not a goal I've ever worked toward, but a "wow, that would be cool" kind of goal. I was a literature major in college, and have always enjoyed any bit of writing that has come along. I did a few articles for a wine industry magazine years ago, and really liked seeing my words in print. I also love public speaking, and I've done a lot of it in business over the years.

So remember that natural "pause point" I mentioned earlier about my career? I have loved the 23 years spent selling wine, but I have been ready to do something else for a while, and COVID has shut down the majority of the distribution channels for wine sales. That sudden unemployment, coupled with the enormous amount of time I have committed to treating a teenager with anorexia, has presented me with a "what's next?" moment. I love writing and have been keeping a journal on my laptop for 10 years that is now 50+ pages long. Every time I write, I feel great not only when I am doing it, but I feel even better afterward. Writing is therapy for me, it gets my feelings and thoughts out, and it forces me to analyze and accept things. I put issues to bed, but I also know that I have a record of how I thought and felt.

I needed to write this book about M's disorder and journey. I needed to write about my struggles, about our unbelievable-if-you've-never-lived-through-this stories. I needed to get all this fear and anxiety out. But I also wanted a record of it, as I didn't want this to fade into our family history. If you are reading this right now, if you are living through something similar, I believe you will feel better if you share your experience. Talk to someone, write it down, sing about it. You may not know it about yourself, but you cannot keep this kind of an experience with a loved one bottled up. If you do, it will hurt you now and in the long run.

All of which also speaks to the bigger picture of taking care of yourself. Like any crisis in your life, the instinct to jump in to fix something or take care of someone can very strong. It's easy to forget about the effects on you, the caretaker. Treating a child with an eating disorder is 24/7/365. It takes years. I feel lucky that M isn't bulimic, one who vomits up after eating. That means I only have to be with her for five meals a day, instead of five meals plus an additional hour after each meal to ensure that she doesn't purge the medicine that is food. But her disorder is on my mind nonstop since I must constantly shop and meal-plan day after day. I have to continually prep favorite foods, while lobbying for and presenting new foods. I have to sit and stare at her while she eats. I must make sure she doesn't hide food. I have to check her afterward: bra and pants and shoes. (Trust me, she's Houdini when it comes to hiding food.) And all this has dragged my strength and happiness and stability down to levels I never thought possible.

I am lucky that I have Tina to help me treat M, but she also works full time and has a work life where she can find other areas of focus. My role as primary caregiver means I have to find time away and outlets that give me a spiritual boost and a break. We started FBT in November, so the weather initially kept us inside. As spring and the heat started arriving, I could sometimes grab a five-hour round of golf with some friends. That was a huge relief to play my usual terrible golf and have a couple of cocktails outside and not have to worry about feeding M. The best activity for me, though, is cycling. I've been at it for 20+ years, having done two San Francisco to Los Angeles charity rides, a couple dozen regular and metric centuries, and tons of training rides with Tina and friends. So when it comes to getting out and away, cycling is key for a few reasons. It physically moves me very far in a small amount of time. A 20-25 mile ride gets me out in the hills, to the next couple of towns over, all in less than 2 hours. Also, the high cardio brings out a lot of sweat and a lot of endorphins. And finally, it is great time inside my head to figure things out.

Peter Sagal brilliantly talked about this in his book *The Incomplete Book of Running*. He shared how the pure act of running, without earphones, without music, books on tape, or podcasts helped him release his negative emotions. He advocated for being in the moment, hearing your own breathing, feeling the cadence of your steps. You are forced to address all the thoughts and ideas that have been building up in the back of your mind, but maybe get ignored because you always are focused on the "now" and consuming other content from a phone or computer or TV. There is so much processing that your brain does in the background, trying to figure things out, that you have to give your brain a chance to spit back the results for you to consider. By following Peter's advice, I started arbitrarily writing sentences and then paragraphs and then pages of this book in my head while I rode. All before I even knew I would write a book.

When Tina and I started FBT around the end of November 2019, we both needed time away from M daily, and she from us, because of the tension and arguments. All of what you have read about in this book was happening behind one closed front door and under one roof. It was where we lived, ate, slept, worked, and treated anorexia. At that early point, Mason (our lovable, 160-pound dog) had no idea that he was about to become a therapy tool. Tina and I would alternate taking "Mr. Large" on 4–5 mile walks, and then we started taking the walks together. It was our time to talk away from M, to complain and to vent, but also to recap and to strategize. If you are treating a child with an eating disorder, be it through facility-based or FBT, and you have a partner, you need consistent and private communication time together. You have to be aligned about that night's dinner and snack, the next day's calorie increase, or which food you are going to introduce that week. These planning sessions, and the relief of knowing you are in the cone of silence, will help you in ways similar to how I describe writing. If you are treating a loved one alone and have no one to walk with, walk anyway. Walking is a slow and peaceful way to move. It forces you to look at small things, things that will take your mind off the demon at home. But it is also your time to evaluate, plan and move on.

Tina went back to work and off FMLA in February 2020, and even during the COVID shutdown, she worked full-time on calls and video meetings from home. M was maintaining her weight and eating pretty well and was starting to move into new topics with her therapist beyond eating: body image, self-confidence, and OCD side effects. So M and I (the unemployed guy) started walking Mason every morning after breakfast, and we unknowingly created a safe space for her to share her thoughts and feelings. She didn't always open up, and I learned not to pry, but she would tell stories about her time in rez, or even ask about new foods. I made it a place to share with her things about my life or explain how random things worked in the world: mortgage refinancing, wine making, warranties. She seemed to like it, and I reveled in having time that was not focused on eating. To have M be herself, gossip about her friends, say that she wanted to recover and eat new things, it almost made me cry a dozen times.

Our FBT routine ran straight into the COVID-19 shelter-in-place order, which was fine because we were used to being home. But the order was bad timing because M had finally gotten back into school in early January 2020 after missing the fall semester, back to seeing her friends, and back to lacrosse. She was a rare sophomore to make the varsity lacrosse team, and all of these distractions and achievements were taking focus off the demon. But now, being at home with nothing to do and no one to see, having had her recently hard-won milestones taken away from her, she had little else to focus on except having to eat and obsess about how many calories were in everything. Isolation, in general, is bad for anyone with mental disorders, but it has an even more debilitating effect on folks with anorexia because it creates a hyper focus on the one thing they need and yet fear the most…with no relief.

There were times when that hyper focus made M really salty to me about everything. Of all people on Earth, I can take any amount of shit and resistance, because I dish it out so much. So please understand that the deflation, the depression, anxiety and partial anger I would feel had to do with my expectations versus the actual progress being made. I gave up my career and my normal life, and I did those willingly and lovingly, because I wanted to help M get better. But when she insulted everything I said, and started to again fight about food portions, started to insist on more food control, started to argue for lower calorie food…all of that was a huge "no progress being made here" sign. I could take the shit and give up my own life for a year or two, but show me that you are changing. Show me that I can feel like the hill below our feet is starting to flatten out. Let me feel that all this is worth it. Let me feel that you are getting better, that you are changing and getting stronger. Maybe you are, but at times I didn't see it and I felt like I was taking a lot of punches for nothing.

There were always bad weeks and backslides. But their existence all the more reinforced that I needed to get out on my bike or with my golf clubs to get a break. I needed to see bits of my own positive life and not get swallowed up by the demon. And as I write all of this, I am starting to feel better. Articulating these words above has helped me see how her backslides fit into the longer narrative. And now I have a record of it to learn from when I read this again later on.

Chapter 8

Just a Matter of Thyme

So much of how and what you prep and cook for your eating disorder patient is sleight of hand, but out in the open. Huh? What I mean is that FBT is meant to be honest and collaborative, with the aim of ultimately turning over control of food prep and eating to the patient. The patient needs to feed themselves and defy the demon. Ride without training wheels, swim without floaties. But the truth is that during weight restoration, and long into weight maintenance, you as the food maker have to develop a Batman utility belt of tricks to get calories into, and keep calories in, a kid who does not want to eat or gain weight. So, fuck the demon, get that kid sober and their weight restored at all costs. The sooner he or she gets sober and re-fed, the sooner there will be a clear mind to address the mental battle of getting rid of the eating disorder demon. This is the ongoing balance of the battle on the two fronts of "weight" and "state."

Dr. Aspen just the other day shared with us how one of her 7th grade eating disorder patients described trying to eat enough food to achieve weight restoration while the demon of anorexia fights against that.

"You have to kill all the bunnies on Earth just to save it" is what eating feels like to that kid suffering from anorexia. It's that hard for people with eating disorders to eat, even though it has to be done and they know it is the only path to recovery. Eating enough to put back on all that weight, eating at all, makes Sisyphus' rock-pushing gig look easy. They have to do that which they loath and fear the most, at bionic levels, to get better, all the while suffering the voice of the demon that enslaved them to begin with. Weight restoration is hell, it's beyond most people's ability to comprehend. These kids have to eat… a lot…all the time…and watch their weight go up and their thighs get bigger, and their chins get softer…and they can't hide food or throw up. And for hours after every meal, they have to hear the voice of the demon in their head scream at them and create an anxiety cocktail with a depression chaser that keeps them up all night, or makes them run away, or makes them cut themselves. Sounds awesome, right?

So how are we going to play our part of hard-ass foe to the demon, or be the "Cook in Chief," knowing that our patient is going to resist and hate whatever we plate in front of them, all the while trying to make it easier on both them and us in pursuit of the bigger goal of weight gain? It is thyme to start deceiving.

I have already talked about how I made M's eggs. So, let's drill down on thyme. It's a simple herb, readily available and cheap. It tastes really good and pretty much goes with anything. The point is, find your "shiny thing." Something for your patient to see or pay attention to, instead of what you are really putting in the dish. Thyme, chives, basil, whatever. It lends great flavor, but it's small and non-threatening, and has no calories. When you add it to eggs that are jacked up with Benecal and heavy whipping cream, your kid only sees the tasty herb. Visual stimuli are very powerful and can make our other senses doubt themselves. "Why are these eggs so rich and flavorful?" gets muted by "Wow, lots of thyme in here."

Here's another meal hack I made up. I found that Campbell's makes a Creamy Tomato Soup in a plastic single serving bowl that has 300 calories. Nice start for a lunch. If you warm that soup up slowly, and get it hot, you can add either a Benecal or a big spoonful of chicken fat and melt that in. Make sure to then boil the soup, then bring the temperature down, then boil it again, then bring it down. The surface of the soup coagulates and then kind of burns, leaving dark red & rippled solid pieces. When you serve the soup in a bowl, sprinkle thyme and crack fresh black pepper on the surface. Make sure there's a piece of toast with either avocado or cream cheese, or plain, depending on where you are with your kid's calorie plan. The point is, the thyme and pepper and burnt surface pieces will easily hide any non-combined Benecal or chicken fat.

Let's get into animal fat. I've mentioned earlier in this book that I find the value of fat calories to be superior. Our kids need carbs and proteins and sugars, but fat has staying power and adds pounds that are harder to burn. I heavily suggest becoming a meat roaster and pit master, a lover of all dead animals that become food for people. This is because animal fat can land bigger punches in the weight gain battle than any other source of fat. At least once a week, I roast 2 full chickens in the oven. Simplest thing in the world. I brine them a day ahead of time for flavor and moisture retention. Once drained, dried, and brought to room temperature, I slather in olive oil and rub it with seasoning, roast for 90 minutes and then these two birds come out of the oven and sit for about an hour. I take the time to break down the white and dark meat, completely scraping all the meat off the carcass...and capturing all the fat and juice that has rendered out into the pan or onto the cutting board. I make sure all of that liquid is poured over the meat in the Tupperware, and it settles nicely at the bottom and coagulates in the fridge. When I go to heat up chicken for M, in goes chicken fat. When I make tomato soup, in goes chicken fat. When we make long grain rice, in goes chicken fat. I just looked up "one tablespoon chicken fat calories" and am happy to report that there are 115 calories in there. I know that you can easily bury two tablespoons into a lot of portions that find their way to your child's plate. That's 230 fat calories you didn't have before. Do that for 8-12 months and know that you have found a Cold War Dead Drop strategy for weight gain that the enemy never knew was happening.

Since you have to ensure that new foods get introduced to your child, along with just volume feeding, work off of your chicken success with other meats. Skirt steak is easier than chicken: sprinkle with salt and pepper, sear on very high heat on side one for 3-4 minutes, turn it over and immediately cover with a high arching lid to sear and convect for another 2-3 minutes for medium rare. Make sure to immediately put the steak into a bowl with foil over the top. After all the steak has rested and cooled, you will have a great lake of jus on the bottom of that bowl. Not as thick nor coagulated as the chicken fat, but you can add that to all sorts of cooking steps that call for broth. And since skirt steak has a nice high fat content, a serving portion that is equivalent to your kids' usual chicken volume will add even more calories.

Plenty of you know your way around food and kitchens, so I ask that you all please embrace the collective concept of animal fats. Render them, collect them, use them. Plus, the more you introduce meats to your child (with all due respect to any vegetarians or vegans reading this), the more successful you will be in adding dense calories to their bodies. (Do not get stuck on some bullshit like commercial frozen chicken parts, there are no meaningful calories there). Another great approach is ground meats. I go to a butcher with plenty of different meats in the case, and they will happily grind anything short of my shopping cart for me. I started out using ground dark meat turkey. Then I started mixing in ground dark chicken, ground pork, ground veal and ground beef. When I cooked them, I would sprinkle in lots of salt, pepper, and thyme, and then I would save the fat that was rendered in the pan. Ground lamb is very distinctive, but when served with a pea puree (frozen peas, garlic, mint, olive oil, salt & pepper whipped in a food processor) M was willing to try it. And in the end, do not always offer to name what you are serving. If asked, it's turkey. Or chicken. Whatever. During refeeding, it's war and the demon can believe whatever you tell it.

I also grow tomatoes during the summer and make my own sauce. Sounds pure and vegetarian to an ED patient. But it also has a ton of olive oil in it and can be made during the winter with canned San Marzanos. The point is, make that and pour it over ground "whatever meat Dad combined." It is a great way to get more fat into your kid.

Bacon fat is another little gem that you can easily file away and access at a moment's notice. We don't cook a lot of bacon in our house, it's usually only on a weekend if we have guests over. So I would cook up a whole package when I knew M would be gone for a couple of hours. Even more specifically, I would cook it outside on the BBQ so there would be no smell in the house.

You will need to drain the bacon grease from the pan into an empty soda can. It's amazing how if you use a standard can opener on a soda can, the top comes off nice and clean. In goes the clear liquid fat, you put it in the fridge for an hour, and then presto! You have nice white solid fat. Keep it hidden in a drawer or cabinet where your kid does not look. For all of the obvious times you can throw it in a pan or pot when warming savory foods, please also consider the basic piece of bread-to-become-toast. I have advocated before that getting your ED kid into burned and well-cooked food is a great tactic during weight restoration, so make sure that well-toasted bread is part of that thinking. Spread a healthy amount of bacon fat on bread before you put it into a toaster, toaster oven, or broiler. The fat soaks into the burned bread. But remember, sleight of hand and misdirected vision is key. That piece of bread is going to have avocado, or cream cheese, or ranch dressing spread on it... and then garlic salt on top of that. Then you put on a bunch of cut up ham and turkey. (Chop lunch meat into small pieces instead of layering whole pieces on a sandwich. Chopped up, and then pressed together between bread, you can get a lot more than 2 or 3 obvious slices of meat into this sandwich. Slices that have lots of fat and protein.) And there is your sandwich full of fat, and I dare anyone to discern the bacon.

Smoothie bowls are the bullshit rallying cry of the "let's be healthy, I wanna be skinny, I'm ok and not anorexic, no I don't have an eating disorder, I follow smart eaters on social media" young kids who make their own food. They pretend that throwing 28 calories of frozen fruit in a blender with ice and 0.3 ounces of protein powder and then eating it out of a pint glass or bowl is a "meal." Sure, and my Cal Bears have the best Rose Bowl record in the Pac 12.

This modest, but potentially significant, reliance on smoothies and bowls could be a warning sign of a kid who is restricting calories, because these "meals" are so nutritionally hollow and yet yield such a high volume. M lived on these for a while right before she fell off the anorexia cliff. I actually believed at the time that she was getting enough calories, but once she was diagnosed and put into recovery, the almighty smoothie became a desperate trojan horse that her affliction would offer up as a meal. M felt that if she could make a smoothie for a snack, all would be good. Right? No. I kid you not, here is what she felt was a fucking snack: 5 frozen strawberry pieces, 2 frozen mango pieces, ice, "very little" protein powder, and lots of water. Mice would starve to death on that. Seriously?

Here is how I hijacked M's smoothie. According to FBT rules, the parent preps and the patient eats. So, she would go so far as to put her 7 pieces of fruit in the blender and then leave the room, supervised by Tina. My version, and I told her, was to add a bit of soy milk. Odd that my wrist didn't comply with my mouth, so lots of soy milk. And a big dollop of heavy whipping cream. Plus, two big scoops of protein powder. And of course, a Benecal. But where is the "thyme" here, Kev? I knew that she loved orange flavor, in the form of the water flavoring called "Meo." A solid squirt of that turned the smoothie into Chernobyl glowing goop, so now I had my smoke screen of color to throw her off.

I initially had to crank up the blender, because the ice was still holding form. At some point, I had to add water to thin it out. What is happening is the formation of an orange sherbet type of drink, oddly enough. The only timer I had to abide by is the heavy whipping cream: I didn't want to over crank this thing to the point where the cream starts to become whipped.

In the end, the final product is icy, bright orange, light and highly acidic. A bit creamy if you look for it, but that's explained away by the "small" addition of soy milk. The nuclear color alone is the best shiny thing ever. And we even got her to add shaved coconut on top. Best as I can remember, this mid-afternoon concoction went for 700+ calories… as a snack. And she loved it. Remember, it's light and bright and fruity. But play with it until you find the right formula.

For all the misery you go through treating an eating disorder patient, you have to embrace the twisted thinking of finding the fun of the revenge tactics in this war. You are stuck in it to win it, and since you will readily discover that initially honesty is not the most effective policy, you may as well get sneaky and land a bunch of hidden blows.

Chapter 9
5150, 5151… Whatever it Takes

I was raised by a father who started his law enforcement career in the San Jose, California Police Department, and who then went on to new agent's class in the FBI at Quantico. He taught me to shoot guns in the basement range of the Federal Building and at the outdoor ranges up in the canyons. I learned that there are two things that you say during a traffic stop: "Yes Officer" or "No Officer."

The point is that I take all law enforcement officers seriously. I feel that anyone who swears an oath as an officer and willingly puts their lives on the line to protect others—I have all the respect in the world for them. These folks are calm and have nerves of steel. Therefore, I believe that whenever someone with a badge and gun is called and shows up, shit is serious. And there are consequences.

I have mentioned elsewhere in this book about having to call the cops on M twice. Those were some of the hardest things in the world I have ever done, and that process slammed reality into my face. I made the decision to call the police with Tina in panicked moments full of fear and unknown facts. Hearing dispatchers on the other end of the phone quickly assess the validity and severity of our issues, and then send officers to our location, made us see that anorexia was going to drag us through more parts of hell than we thought possible.

The first time we called the police was when M ran away on a Thanksgiving trip out of town. We had just broken the news to M that we were pulling her from the PHP program because she was slipping backwards so badly. We also said that, while we were "this close" to sending her to the ERC in Denver to increase her level of care, we instead would be holing up with her at home indefinitely until FBT got her weight restored and put her on the road to recovery. Shocker that she bolted, right?

We were in a small town, so we called both the City Police and County Sheriff. They were amazingly responsive and accommodating, and they put a couple of hours into looking for her. It was raining and cold outside, and we had no idea where to look. M was never found by the officers, but she came home on her own a couple of hours later, in the dark and pouring rain. She said she went to hide to scare us, to get back at us, to fuck with us. One of the officers spoke to her to assess her health, safety, and sanity, and ultimately left her with us. He did, though, try to put a scare into her and told her not to do it again.

The second time we called the cops was a couple of months later. We had found some early success with FBT, and M had put back on about 80% of the weight she needed. And though the going was rocky, we were moving forward and making progress. She was back to school, she was close to weight restoration, and she was trying hard to put herself in a position to go out for Varsity Lacrosse. These are all huge "wins," huge realities that just months ago were fantasies and "fuck it, my life is over, I'll never get those back." But then one day, we had our weekly session with Dr. Aspen, and M's weight was close to a "restoration" number that M felt was way too high, and this made her lash out at us. She wanted to slow down the weight gain, and thus declared that drinking milk at any meal was no longer acceptable. She instantly became very dark and angry. She shut down and blacked us out.

This story may sound like it is just about drinking milk. So, I need to make this point very clear, as it is a recurring roadblock that leads to conflict. Eating disorders find a patch of grass to fight over and they dig in for the fight of a lifetime. In this case, it was drinking milk with meals. "Who the FUCK drinks milk with every meal? That's crazy, no way, game over, I dare you to try and make me," the demon roared. You cannot back down, but you also cannot believe this is about drinking milk. This is about the disorder seeing its own demise, seeing that you are making progress on it. That fucker has been throwing buckets and boxes out the back window of a speeding escape car as you chase it, trying to slow you down. This is just an episode where the disorder pulls the car over, squats behind the open driver's door, and starts shooting at you. You have to hold your ground, fight over that patch of grass, until the disorder drives off again knowing that you will never give up the pursuit.

That night at dinner after the Dr. Aspen appointment, Tina had to be gone, so I was flying solo and served M her usual glass of milk with dinner. With quite a proclamation, she threw that glass across the floor toward the wall in the same angle you would skip a flat rock on a lake. I stayed calm, as I kind of knew something like this was going to happen. And while it's a bitch to clean up milk and shattered glass across two rooms with a combination of tile and carpet, I kept my cool. Granted, the dogs yelped and ran to the front room to hide, but I didn't make any grand gestures or protests.

After the episode, I poured another glass of milk and told her she was required to drink it. She ate the entirety of her dinner, but then ran off to her room screaming and locked the door. I executed the FBT playbook by going to her door, calm and reassuring, and told her that she needed to finish her milk. But I also modified my strategy by employing patience and by not going hard core on her. She was super spun up, the demon was terrorizing her, there was no way I was going to use brute force to win at that moment. I walked away.

When Tina got home later, we talked about what happened, and I assumed that by that time M had probably cried herself to sleep. We left her alone and went to bed, and we both agreed to serve her a bigger glass of milk the next morning.

When the next morning arrived, M came downstairs looking like she had been at a fraternity party all night. She had obviously wrestled with sleep, she had been beaten up by the demon, and she was trying to hold together her resolve to fight. We presented her with breakfast and poured the milk. And lo and behold, here came the battle. She screamed and threatened us, she threatened the dogs, she unloaded everything she had thought about all night. Then she reared up and smashed the glass of milk against the floor and wall. She then ran screaming out of the room. Breakfast remained uneaten.

There had been a point a few weeks earlier when Dr. Aspen had told us during our session, in front of M, that if she acted in a manner that threatened anyone's safety, we needed to call the police. It was shocking, and it was something that I was still unsure of at the time. You know that scene in a lot of random crime movies, when a weaker character is handed a gun by some badass character, and is instructed to "use it when the time comes"? You know that look on the weaker person's face, like "You're fucking with me, right? I'm not gonna shoot this thing."

That was me when Dr. Aspen dropped that ultimatum on us about the importance of calling the police, even though we had already called them on M back in November. That first call was because M ran away, not because she was a danger. Well now, M was a danger. And we also needed a "BAM" moment, a course correction, a wake-up call to how bad this was becoming. So, we called the County Sheriff, and told the dispatcher that our daughter had a mental disorder, that she was verbally threatening us and the animals, and that she had acted out violently twice in the last 12 hours. We hung up and told M they were on the way

When the two officers showed up about 15 minutes later, it turned out to be the actual Sheriff herself, along with a veteran deputy. They came in and I expected to have to describe everything, to help them figure out what to do. Oh no, they had this. They had seen this before, and they knew how this whole scenario was going to play out.

Just to be clear, 5150 is the California law code for the temporary, involuntary psychiatric commitment of individuals who present a danger to themselves or others due to signs of mental illness. It may be the last resort for parents dealing with situations like this, or it may be an escalation lever to pull. Either way, that was what we were doing.

The Sheriff told M to come downstairs, she did not ask. M came down from her room and went to the couch in the living room and she balled up. She had her arms wrapped around her bent knees and she had her face slammed into her kneecaps. She was hyperventilating and her face was red and stretched tight. The demon was seeing what kind of gun we had brought to this knife fight. The Sheriff asked M a series of questions that sounded like hostage rescue negotiations, this woman knew how to talk someone down. And also, like a great lawyer on cross examination, she got M to admit to violent and dangerous behavior. The Sheriff started easy, just telling M to make all of this go away by eating breakfast and going to school. Just fucking eat, right?

I can't remember M's exact comeback, but let's just say it was really disrespectful by normal standards, let alone when said to an officer of the law. Then, the weirdest thing happened. I've already talked about my respect for police officers, and their ability to stay calm and bring law and order to chaos. Well, the deputy was still standing across the room, and he looked about my age. Easy to believe he had teenage kids. He lost his shit. Not diplomatically, or empathetically, but full rage cage. He yelled, "Shut the fuck up. I went through this shit with my daughter last year. You are not going to do this to your parents."

After that outbreak, the Deputy and the Sheriff then landed the knockout punch on M: they told her to either get up and to eat all her breakfast, plus milk, or they were taking her out of here on a stretcher. She would be handcuffed to that stretcher. The ambulance would take her to the hospital. Not Stanford's eating disorder unit, but the county hospital. She would stay there for three days until they said she was ok to come back and try this conversation again. Mic down.

There was a lot of silence, there were a lot of tears, and there was the look of terror and fear in M's face as she had to break from the demon to save herself. She went to the kitchen, and she demanded that we all leave her alone, which we all did except for me, who sat and watched her eat. FBT rules still applied. Tina talked in the front hall with the Sheriff and the deputy for about 15 minutes. Once the air in the house started to thin out a bit, and we all knew what direction this was going, the Sheriff came back into the kitchen to say goodbye to M and me. M raised her middle finger and told the County Sheriff to go fuck herself. And while I was trying to grasp that moment, the Sheriff came back with a pretty solid verbal backhand, something along the lines of "you can pull that shit with your parents, but I'm the Sheriff of this county, you will treat me with respect and you better hope that I don't have to come back." I am paraphrasing, but that's pretty close.

After M finished her breakfast, including milk, we all got ready and we took her to school. I loved signing her in late to the attendance office and seeing the part of the sheet that said, "Reason for being late." I'm pretty sure I left it blank.

Tina and I were paranoid all morning about what we would hear from her or from the school. Would M take off, lose her shit in class, go crazy on campus? Almost worst, we had to meet her at lunch in the car in the parking lot and watch her eat. How would that go?

I could go on and on with this chapter, but this is a great way to sum it up. M didn't go nuts at school, though later she described it to us as the worst day of her life, having to walk in and out of classes and keep her sobs to herself. She came out to our car at lunch that day and ate all of her lunch without incident. She then came home that day after school, ate snack, and did homework. She also came down for dinner that night. She ate the food we served and drank the milk we poured. The BAM moment had worked. The demon knew we were fighting to win. M knew we were willing to make her unhappy and uncomfortable in order to beat this eating disorder. It was also a small numbing of Tina's and my fear toward the demon, and I think we came to the same conclusion any combatant comes away with after surviving a battle. The war was not over, but we'd gone to the brink in this one battle, and we had all come back together. I'll never know how truly horrible I made my daughter feel that day, but I'll do it again if I have to. Whatever it takes.

Chapter 10
Narcos

Another critical medical professional you will need in this journey is a psychiatrist, who is also a highly trained therapist for your child, but one who can prescribe medicine. And I'm not talking about anti-inflammatories or blood thinners. I am talking about drugs for your kid's head that will help calm the demon's voice or relax the terrors that are driving the eating disorder.

There is a tremendous amount of debate and discourse about vaccinating and medicating ourselves, let alone our children. In the case of eating disorders, there is a great amount of anxiety and terror that is ruling a child's mind. One way to ease that psychological roadblock is the use of various anti-anxiety medications. The correct medication, at the correct dosage, can lower the temperature and the noise and the resistance in a child's mind and allow them to eat with greater ease as they try to get refed and sober. The correct medication can also mean that a child will put up less of a fight when receiving therapy. Thus, the correct medication can facilitate winning the battle with both "weight" and "state."

The decision to use medication is unique to each patient and each family. Tina and I felt that if M had diabetes, we would use insulin to allow her to eat and live out her life. If M had a broken leg, we would get her crutches so that she could walk and be independent. We took the same perspective with anorexia, in that we felt that medication would make the demon in her head weaker and she would be able to eat and recover in a more comfortable manner. There were some early adjustments and changes, and even just recently at two plus years, her medication was slightly increased and it made a huge difference.

We are very aware of the fact that many of these medications, and very specifically the one that M is using, present their own set of issues that must be overcome. M had to be on her medication for a few months before the benefits started to manifest and she could feel less anxiety. Also, her medication worked better if she ate more and carried more weight. Plus, once her body was acclimated to the medicine, if she skipped a day, she would get immediate uncomfortable side effects. She describes the most prominent side effect as a "brain zap," where streaks of light go across her vision and her emotions are more volatile.

In the long term, there will also be quite a lengthy offramp when she no longer needs the medicine, and we wean her off of it. Right now, we are trading off the fact that her body is completely acclimated to having her medicine act like the aforementioned insulin or crutches for her anorexia. It is allowing her to eat regularly with less and less mental stress, and it is buying her time for her body to rebuild and for her mind to move on permanently from the disorder. Once she is in control of eating and is no longer at risk of slipping back into dangerous behaviors, once she is strong enough to keep the eating disorder at bay with her own strength, we will start to slowly pull back the insulin & crutches. We are willing to deal with that issue later in life, as we see a very safe, slow, and medically monitored withdrawal from a prescription drug is worth the benefit it is providing now.

You have to find out the facts about medications that could help ease your child's struggle, and also whether or not your child is a suitable candidate for them. This decision is between you, your spouse, and your child. It's always a good idea to talk to other parents who have been faced with this same decision, but ultimately your child has their own specific needs. This is a terrorizing time for your child, and you need to consider everything that might help them.

Chapter 11
I Am a Fraud

This happens all the time, revolving every few days, throughout the weeks and months. I am a fraud. I am writing a book about helping my daughter recover from anorexia, about how I left my job to focus on her, about how I am shoulder-deep in battling the demon and learning the lessons of eating disorders. Yet, I fail all the time. I am not that smart, I am not that strong, and I question why the hell you bought and read this book.

Two days ago, we talked to M about having fish tacos for dinner. It was a great conversation, and she said things like "that sounds good" and "here is how I will make them." All of these are signs of hunger and desire that normal people would ascribe to forthcoming food. Signs and comments that show an evolution for an anorexia sufferer who is moving forward in the journey of accepting food. But when we discussed portions, specifically two corn tortillas per taco instead of one, she dug in. Nope, just one tortilla per taco is all she would have, but she would have more fish. Yes, this would calorically be equivalent, but this is a huge red flag we had to drive at. If she was vehemently avoiding something, we had to take that barrier down. You must recognize this response and this behavior as disorder 101 and you must attack an entire meal over a small point like this.

Our first discussion with M about the fish taco dinner was around noon that day, and you already know what she said. I came back to her midway through the afternoon to help her agree to our plan, but she stuck to her guns. I tried to be good cop, encouraging her, in a time and place away from food, that she could do it. No fucking way, she said. I tried negotiating, saying that she could have one big flour tortilla or two small corn tortillas. Still, according to her, no fucking way.

I talked to Tina about the conversation, looking to see where she and I could agree on a strategy, one that would not set M off in a rage, but Tina held firm to two tortillas. I felt helpless and frustrated, and I said, "Dr. Aspen tells us to empathize with her struggles, but you are pushing for a position she will not accept. I have tried to push our case to M, she refuses, and now you are steadfast in not negotiating. And I am in the middle. Unable to push either solution." See where I am? I have no power, I cannot push either option, and I cannot negotiate with either party. On that day I didn't have the guts to just line up with Tina because I was scared of my daughter. At that moment, I was paralyzed and that familiar, sinking feeling reemerged—the feeling that I was a fraud, totally ineffective in battling this torrential demon.

When dinnertime came around, it turned out that two of M's friends showed up and M did not want to make a scene in front of them. Tina quietly but firmly made M plate two corn tortillas per taco and M quietly ate them with no fight. I stood off to the side and did nothing. Tina was right to push M and make her go further. I was a fraud of a parent who was afraid of the strong will of both my wife and my daughter.

FBT, or any form or treating anorexia, puts you in a position where you have to exert control over the demon. You have to push aside the pushback, you cannot be afraid of the fight, or the shots fired at you. You have to move forward, you cannot accept status quo, you have to pull your kid out of the quicksand and out of the jungle. You cannot stay still. But you have to be empathetic, you have to side with your kid, you have to recognize when they are struggling or begging for help. This whole thing is like driving in fog with no lane lines.

This chapter is here for me to say that when presented with a simple meal-ingredient-volume debate, I did not remember nor learn from any of the previous experiences I had been through. I showed none of the strength I thought I had when faced with the thought of getting into a huge fight and then possibly losing a meal's worth of calories. I let too many debates happen in my head between helping my daughter feel better vs pushing my daughter past a stupid impediment put up by the demon. I did not exert the guts and wisdom of someone who had quit his job to help his anorexic daughter. I did not show any of the street cred of someone who thought he could write a book about battling anorexia. In my mind, I had failed. At that moment, I truly was convinced I was a fraud.

Chapter 12
A Trip Around the Sun

Since the beginning of our FBT journey, Dr. Aspen has told M to set up some rewards that she could work toward throughout weight restoration and weight maintenance. She said that M should get something in return for all of the pain and stress she would have to endure. M initially did not do anything with this advice, as she told us that she was more motivated by consequences than rewards. In other words, she would rather avoid a bad thing than get a good thing. But another sign of her winning the battle of the "state" was a change in her thinking on that topic. She started to find other ways of seeing herself as beautiful or attractive that were not weight related. So, she came to us with this question: if she ate dessert once a week, ongoing, could she get her belly button pierced? Dessert would be in addition to night snack, unless the dessert portion was big. We loved the idea, and we couldn't care less about a piercing. If that was her idea of beauty and happiness, and it helped to create better eating habits, so be it.

M started her dessert exercise by eating frozen, chocolate-covered bananas and strawberries. These are not ideal heavyweight sweets, but this whole exercise is like so many other recovery strategies: start with very small steps and have faith that they will lead to big strides. So those four to five little fruit bites soon were joined by three or four small cookies. We never asked or told her about eating dessert, she would just go to the kitchen on her own once a week after dinner and bring them out. And don't see this as us trying to add calories to her, that was not the point. The point was that M, like any of us, will be faced with dessert in life. She will go to a birthday party, she will walk past a bakery, she might date someone with a sweet tooth. She cannot be afraid of occasionally having dessert. It's part of life. One night, she grabbed ten little cookies that you get in a big plastic tub from Trader Joe's. She didn't flinch, she just ate them. Then the next day, unsolicited, she mentioned that eating those ten little cookies wasn't really a big deal. Steps to strides.

About eight weeks into this routine, she asked if she could get the piercing on her "Anniversary." I had mentioned previously to her that the one-year milestone of her being diagnosed and admitted to Stanford Hospital was coming up, and here she was seeing it as something to celebrate. We thought that was a great idea but said that her dessert portions needed to get a little bigger, and she complied.

We decided that since she was put into Stanford Hospital, we would celebrate the day by walking around Stanford Shopping Center. Remember, we're still in the middle of COVID, so there's not a lot to touch and try on. After M and I looked at all the clothes and linens and jewelry in the windows that we didn't buy, I drove her up to the only piercing salon open in the Bay Area during the pandemic. We waited in line in the parking lot for about four hours, and M even did her weekly therapy call with Dr. Aspen from the car while I held our place in line. We also missed her midafternoon snack, but we were determined for a million reasons to go through with this. She was a year into recovery, she was eating dessert, there was a salon open, and all that waiting in line was not going to waste.

Once inside, everything about the last year and the last four hours disappeared. The whole world was simply about getting a cool piercing and letting M feel good about her body. The woman who did the piercing was really cool, had big white hair and a body full of tattoos and piercings. She looked like the perfect person to do the job. She laid M back on a reclined barber's chair and talked her through the process and was very calming. The whole thing took about 20 minutes, and there was no dulling agent or numbing cream, just a very steady hand and a very sharp needle. By 5:30 we were out the door, heading to Safeway to pick up a late snack, and then we were on the road for the hour drive home. With a piece of metal through her stomach. The stomach that a year ago barely held enough food to keep her alive.

A day like that proves so many things to me. Recovery is a long, slow, painful slog through mud and lava. It never ends. But short-term and intense pain in exchange for long-term gain is the strategy that works. Fight the demon head on, inspect what you expect, don't take no for an answer, keep moving forward. If your actions cause the disorder to flare up, you are doing something right. Every conflict with your kid is gut-wrenching, but every time you face and beat the demon you have gotten closer to killing it. There will be gains and unexpected victories that accompany the backslides. All the small steps will turn into long strides if you keep pushing it. Even just putting the one-year date out there as an arbitrary goal created a reason to celebrate.

This day also reminded me about priorities. All I care about for M is that she eats and recovers. I want her to be free from this disorder, I want her to be happy. Piercings, or even odd haircuts and hair coloring and ripped jeans and makeup, those are not things to stress over as a parent. Who cares, especially if these things make them happy while they are suffering through the mental battle of a lifetime. Do you all remember what you wanted to do and look like as a teenager, and you didn't even have a mental disorder? Becoming a healthy and happy young adult who survives this kind of trauma will be an outcome that is worth whatever cosmetic adjustments they want.

It sucks to have to constantly fight your kid over food and weight, to watch them eat and pat them down after meals, to search their rooms for hidden food and to keep them out of the bathroom for an hour after meals. Conversely, it feels so good, so normal, so nice to be the fun parent and give them a "yes" once in a while. Allowing your eating disordered teenager an indulgence, one that in normal times would make them happy, is multiplied by a factor of five when they are living in the depths of anger and anxiety and pain and fear. This ray of sunshine into their jail cell also reminds them of a normal world where they want to live. It reminds them that there is a world where fun can be had and piercings can make you feel beautiful and confident.

The long-term gains that we are living with as I write this chapter are these. M preps and plates 85% of her meals. M will remind me if I forgot to get out her juice, or when her Zoloft prescription is almost out, or if we need more avocados. M has given up her exercise when her weight drops as an acknowledgment of needing to hold more calories. M is asking for a variety of different foods and is asking to try some of her old favorites. We eat at restaurants without seeing the menu ahead of time. M has admitted that she is starting to still be hungry after some meals and is working up the courage to ask for seconds. She realized the other day that she hadn't told me to fuck off in over two weeks. She is slowly separating from the demon; she is being just M on her own for hours at a time. She is becoming strong and returning to being our little girl.

But there is also a danger of complacency when you and your child start to turn a few corners. We have seen M be so positive around food for a couple of months now, and her anger is starting to disappear. But she also had a modest backslide about a month ago, and suddenly we could not find six pounds. Where did they go? And though we weighed her every week, she still was holding onto the trick of water-loading to boost her weight and was hiding the fact that she just wanted to cruise along under her healthy weight.

When we finally discovered the ruse, and she finally agreed to doing weigh-ins at face value, we were hit by the fact that this never ends. We had temporarily blinded ourselves with "so much good news and progress" that we didn't see her getting skinnier.

We are back to "gain" mode, and it has to be at least a pound a week, and we need to go unearth those six pounds. M had a bit of a flareup at us initially about the amount of weight she had to put back on, demanding that the goal weight number was "never part of the deal," whatever that means. The flareup scared me, and actually really punched me in the gut and made me really stressed. Dr. Aspen calls these moments "extinction bursts" because the demon is trying to go down swinging. But as with all things going extinct, the demon's strength is limited. By the next day, M and I talked about how to up her meal plan and we agreed that we are on a mission to get back to "maintenance" mode. She came back from being told what to do by the demon, she was ready to hit a number and not rig her weight.

I was reminded that there will always be backslides, that I need to be vigilant, and that M's anger cycles are getting shorter. I was also reminded that there is a happy girl in there, who is desperately trying to make progress in how she sees herself and how she wants to act. And that happy girl probably found a small amount of strength by looking down at her belly button piercing, and then smiling to herself about how great she looked, and then knowing that she could keep moving forward with recovery.

Chapter 13
Weapons of War

Looking back on this epic slog through hell, and as I write this I am still deep in it, I find the need to share the inventory of tips and tricks that I have amassed. There are so many workarounds and backups that I have invented, copied, or improved upon (and God knows how many more you readers have) that I wanted to create a bit of a field guide for folks new to this fight.

I have had a second refrigerator in my garage for fourteen years now, and I will never go back to only having the one in the kitchen. Extra storage and cooling space is useful to everyday life, let alone having kids, let alone liking to entertain a lot, let alone having a kid with anorexia. But it also must not be accessible. It must be locked. Yes, you have to get a lock that seals to the door and requires a key. We keep one key in my desk in the office, and another one hidden in the garage. M knows there is no access to this fridge, so she knows that this is an armory designated to killing her demon. We not only keep backups of her go-to foods, but that is where I keep the heavy whipping cream for the F-U eggs. I also store all the rendered animal fat from chicken and steak and pork and veal when I need to deploy it in any manner.

It is also where I store the drinks that she pours herself. Why would you do that, Kevin? Because, for a kid who knows they have to drink the milk or juice that is in the fridge, what do they do late at night when you're asleep? They water it down. And then they pour it out into a glass front of you and drink it with gusto to make you feel like you're winning when you are not. M went so far as to open all the tetra packs of protein shakes, empty them, and refill with water. She would then put on quite a show of having her snack by getting one out of the fridge and guzzling it down. My point is, lock up anything that your kid can secretly adulterate on the altar of the demon.

Also get a thick, black magic marker and black out all calorie labels on food you bring into the house from the store. Or use scissors to cut out parts of labels. Now the shitty part of doing this extra work is that any kid can look up the calories of anything in your cupboards on the internet. Nonetheless, blacked out calories and fat will signal to her that she will have to work harder. And it's another sign to the demon that you are minding the details. (Note: as of this publishing, M now cuts the labels off food herself.)

Don't be afraid to switch packaging. I buy the tortillas that are 230 calories each, and somehow, they fit nicely into another brand's bag that says 110 calories. The real tortillas, with backups of the higher calorie ones, are kept in the locked garage fridge, before they are transferred to the fake packaging in the kitchen fridge. You can even pour higher calorie milk into lower calorie packaging, one that has the nutrition label blacked out. And the same logic works by just removing the labels on cans of soup or bottles of cranberry juice. The kid doesn't know the brand and will only see the vessel.

Speaking of packaging, kids with eating disorders are unscrupulous and devilish. They will stay up all night or get up early or fake going out just to dig into what you are buying, storing, and feeding to them. You will find many times when you have to hide labels and vessels of what was served instead of just simply tossing them out. It's one thing to constantly take out the garbage and recycling to the side yard where the kids are less inclined to dumpster dive. It is another thing to have serious hiding places and disposal protocols. Whenever we used Benecal in M's eggs, the plastic cup was rinsed and cleaned, the foil top was crushed to hide all writing, and that was shoved into the cup with a tissue, and then the whole thing was wrapped in a paper towel before being shoved down the shaft of the 5 iron inside my golf bag to the bottom, the golf bag I kept inside my travel bag at the back of the garage. Yup, I'm nuts. I would actually say to myself, inside my head, while making the F-U eggs and disposing of the Benecal, "Do not break protocol." Getting caught is the worst thing that I could do for my "Chef" relationship with the girl who barely trusted me to make her food. The point is, you will have to dispose of lots of evidence, so if you're going to do it, go full Ocean's Eleven and do it right. Just remember to dump out your golf bag at the turn while you're getting a drink.

Embrace the caloric density of nuts and seeds. Chia

seeds, for example, are these beautiful, small, black beads, no bigger than one tenth of a grain of rice. They have 140 calories and 9 grams of fat in 2 tablespoons, and these can disappear into a pot of brown wild rice with chicken fat like DB Cooper into the desert, never to be seen or known of again.

You can also make the afternoon snack a very small baggie of mixed nuts. I seriously did the following exercise. I bought separate big bags each of almonds, pistachios, cashews, peanuts, macadamia nuts, sunflower seeds, pine nuts, pecans, whatever. I found that the serving size was usually about 12-16 nuts per each kind. I made piles of one serving of each nut. Then I blended a portion of each kind of nut into joint piles, counting to keep track of calories. I ended up with 5 or 6 piles of equal portions of a mix of each kind of nut, and each pile was 400-600 calories, mostly made up of fat. Once I put each pile into a slightly larger-than-needed Ziploc bag ("Sandwich" size is fine, "Quart" is better) and shook it all into a corner and held the bag at a 45-degree angle, it did not look like a big portion. I paired that bag with an apple or a banana, or glass of juice, and I may hit 550-750 calories in mid-afternoon with little resistance.

Grocery shopping is another huge issue when treating kids with eating disorders. You CANNOT take them to the grocery store. Not at all. Shopping while anorexic is like driving while drunk: no reasonable or safe decisions can be made, and it will only lead to pain. You as the parent must make all the purchases away from prying eyes, pursuant to your refeeding plan, with no influence from the patient. If you bring that kid to the grocery store, you will spend more time fighting off the desperate conniving of the demon for lower calorie and bullshit food. The point is, there is no place in your food shopping and prep for your eating disorder kid during the early stages of refeeding.

There was a point where M started eating a certain cereal and was really happy with it. She actually said that it was fun to be back to eating cereal. So Dr. Aspen suggested we use the tactic of "Chaining" to play off this success. This meant that we suggested another cereal from the same brand or use another brand but with the same flavor. M slowly built up four or five different cereals that she was happy to eat, and this was a huge win for both weight and state, as it kept her eating and broke down rigid resistance to new foods. Take this tactic and apply anywhere that you see a lot of extensions for a food your kid has taken a liking to.

Density is key. I have already extolled the virtues of fat over carbs for the sake of staying power and proportions. But that is true for both during early FBT when the patient is blind to the contents of the meal, but also for later when open honesty is key to the patient prepping their own meals. We just recently had a big weight loss that M admitted to plotting, but she acknowledged the need to correct. We blatantly told her that smaller but more dense food options were coming, and she liked. She knew more eating was required but feared "bigger" meals that would make her uncomfortable. So, no more salads or hummus, here comes eggs or avocado or cream cheese. No more chicken here comes beef. And strangely enough, new cranberry mixed juices showed up that were higher in calories for the same volume.

You also must embrace Green Sauce. Seriously, sounds odd, and there are many different versions, but it rocks. It has avocados and olive oil and pistachio nuts, which are very dense with fat & calories, and yet it tastes so refreshing. It goes with and on everything. It is insane. Do the calorie and fat math on a batch, and then estimate what a portion will do to your kids' calorie intake during a meal. Not to mention, it will become a house favorite for the rest of the non-ED folks. Just blend all this together in a food processor.

- 1 avocado
- 1 cup packed parsley and cilantro leaves (combined)
- 1 jalapeño, ribs and seeds removed
- 2 cloves garlic
- juice of two limes
- ½ cup water
- ½ cup olive oil
- 1 teaspoon salt
- ½ cup pistachios (you can sub other nuts)

As long as your kid does not have a health issue with dairy, please do not allow yourself to go down the nut milk road. All nut milks are made of is water and crushed nuts. And while I have extolled the virtue of nuts for snacks, nut milks do not pack the calorie or fat punch of dairy milk. Why the hell do you think they are so popular with the rest of the world? You need to set the bar for your kid's milk as coming from a cow, and that low-fat to whole milk is good. These calories have more fat and calcium in them, and dairy-based milk is usually easier to find. You do not want to run into a situation out in public where your kid orders a nut milk from a restaurant that does not carry it. That becomes an excuse to not drink and may even lead to a fight. And while later in life, long after recovery has set in, your kid can and will embrace any number of lighter or alternative foods…during the battle of FBT you need to use common and high-calorie foods.

Do you all remember the secret ingredient to the Fuck You Eggs? Benecal. Order it by the case on Amazon. Have it delivered to the red Amazon pick up locker at your local grocery store so it doesn't show up at your house (as the box is labeled on the outside). Hide the small containers in the file drawer with your insurance forms and tax records. Experiment with blending it into different hot or cold dishes. This little boost will help in the early days of weight gain, but you will have to wean off of it as you turn back over control of food to your kid later on.

It really helps to keep a weekly meal journal during the refeeding process, at least for the first three to four months. You may be really overwhelmed by all the moving parts, so keeping a record that you can refer back to can ease your mind. Since you will be preparing three meals and three snacks a day, break each day's section into six areas. Keep it simple, use whatever shorthand works for you. But make sure to list each meal or ingredients that you prepared, then check off whether or not you kid liked it (put up a fight?), whether or not your kid finished it (needed liquid supplement?), and how many calories were ingested. Then total up how many calories you think got into that kid's belly in each day. At the end of the week, add up all seven days of calories and list that next to the amount of weight that was gained or lost over that same period.

One funny side note here to consider is, when looking for a food journal to use, most of them are geared toward helping you LOSE weight. Either overwrite a simple formatted one, make your own, or just use a legal pad.

Which leads me to the whole point of all this feeding and calorie cramming, which is to get weight back on your kid. Weight restoration is the key to being physically sober and the starting point where your child can see and feel their body as it should be. So how do you know when the weight is back on? You need a scale that works well, so don't skimp here. The one from your bathroom and the 1990s is out of whack, plus you need one that keeps records and captures additional metrics. I use Arboleaf and its accompanying app. It records a full panel of metrics for every time that M steps on, such as her body weight, water weight, BMI, body fat, etc. All these metrics can then be seen on a graph over time, showing all the specific weigh-in dates, that I can match against the journal of foods and calories I talked about above. Here is where all the single data points can paint a trend for me to follow. Also, I can share the data with our FBT therapist or eating disorder physician. Finally, it is best to consistently use the same scale throughout refeeding. If you get incorrect or different weight numbers from a different scale at a doctor's office or friend's house, that can seriously throw off a feeding plan and bring down morale even with 1-2 pounds difference.

And of course, none of this planning and plotting is without its enemy. Remember the demon, and don't think for a minute that it is not trying to rig the weigh-in process. A kid with an eating disorder is scared to death to know they are gaining weight, and it makes the demon furious to know it is losing its grip. These kids starved themselves for a variety of reasons, and while they may want to recover, gaining weight is their biggest fear. They are trying to play along and eat, but they are also hiding or spitting up or purging as much food as possible. In order for them to maintain the demon's ruse is to trick the one way of seeing if all this FBT is working, which is the scale.

First of all, the weigh-in is done with your kid wearing the least amount of clothing that can add weight or hide things. M would wear a sports bra, shorts or PJ pants, and no shoes. A boy should be shirtless with shorts. The easiest thing a kid will do is water-load, which is to guzzle lots of water right before the scale comes out. If you make sure the kid goes to the bathroom first, and if you track the water weight metric on your new scale afterward, you should be able to eliminate that trick. Also know that kids will take rolls of coins or fishing weights or shotgun shells and hide them in various body openings. They may hide a variety of high density, yet small shaped, objects in their hair bun or under their armpit or attached to their inner thigh. Just make sure you set very strict rules for weigh-in, and even do pat-downs and inspections, as this is the only way to validate all the hard work you are doing.

I cannot begin to imagine the number of tricks and ideas that all of you have been thinking about or saying out loud. Sharing this kind of information with each other as caregivers of ED sufferers starts to take a bit of the sting out of treatment. What I mean is that, once you make treating eating disorders a group battle or a shared fight, you start to feel that you have ammunition, momentum, and support. Just by laughing about how you are fucking over your kids' demon with another parent can help make one meal or one week feel like winning the war is possible.

Chapter 14

You Made Today Really Hard

This is the part of the book where I may appear to contradict philosophies, strategies, and tactics that I have extolled earlier. Maybe I'm learning and evolving. Maybe this journey goes blindly forward, and around future corners lie things I hadn't expected. This whole odyssey is such a whirlwind, and here is where I have been blown off course.

We are quite a way into FBT at this point, and M is doing things I would never have thought possible. And I have to realize that all of this "progress" is torture for her. She started a while ago with pouring all her own drinks with each meal, and then having to live with drinking all that juice and then facing her demon. I kind of want her to be thinking "See, Demon, I'm taking charge of eating to defeat you. Mom and Dad aren't the only enemies." Next, she started to plate her meals, with our supervision, from an array of food we prepare. And now she is fully going to the cupboards and fridge to collect a variety of food, and completely preparing her breakfast and afternoon snack.

This is epic, and for anyone reading this right now who is stuck early on in treatment and recovery for ED, you may think it impossible. And it was impossible, until it wasn't. Because we just kept at it. But again, along with all this great freedom and control for M comes great responsibility and great consequences. She has to face the demon more and more after she is solely responsible for defying it.

Today is day four or five of M having a fever and sore throat. She has fortunately tested negative for COVID-19, but strep throat or something else is still be lingering. The point is, she is really beat up and mostly in bed, and has asked me to go back to making meals for her. It is super sweet, and it really makes me happy to take care of my little girl, no ED considerations, just a dad who wants to make her meals. What I did today, and what I did not think of, are two things you need to know.

First of all, we decided to stray from the F-U Eggs for lunch this week and try something else. And what sounds better than chicken noodle soup when you are sick? Nothing, so off to the store I went to find a few cans. Of course, I went for the highest calorie soup I could find, still way below the eggs, but soup with some sustenance. When I first served it to her along with some crackers, she liked both and she was happy. So what did I do? What did I fucking do? I went back to the store and got "creamy" chicken noodle soup. I got greedy. I couldn't just think of my daughter, eons into the nightmare of anorexia and days into a 103-degree fever and want to replicate her happiness at a bowl of soup and some crackers that she admitted liking.

Nope, I was stuck in first gear, in no negotiating with terrorists, in no rules in war.

When we served her the creamy version of the soup the next day, M flipped out. She caught it, she knew. I actually was out of the house for a couple of hours on an errand and Tina was left holding the bag of creamy soup. I was called, I was yelled at, I denied everything. But M knew, and yet, she ate. She was pissed and fuming and felt denied justice but knew she had to eat.

She has to live with herself after meals, *she* has to deal with the demon. When she knew that she ate a higher calorie and higher fat meal, then she knew that the consequences would be higher when faced with the demon. When I got home from my errands, she gave me a brief silent treatment, but then laid on me the Acme Anvil from hell. "Dad, you made today really hard." Simply said, but infinite in its implications. She had been happy with that meal yesterday while struggling through a miserable fever. She had been able to get along with that soup and crackers, but then today, I made her miserable.

Now I still believe that any blow to the demon is worth it, but the further along you get into recovery, the more you have to consider your kid's part in the battle. They start to move away from being fully aligned, across the battlefield, with the demon, and they move more to your side of enemy lines. M was starting to do her part to fight the demon, I didn't have to do it all. And remembering that we were trying to strengthen her "state" (of mind), I needed to worry less about the "weight." Yet I let my old habits, though totally valid 5-7 months ago, get the better of me today. I needed to be more aware of her status in this odyssey.

But, part of this moving forward is that my perspective constantly changes, and here is where I am going to turn this chapter around again. Making M uncomfortable and unhappy is, well, part of our job in FBT. The only way to shake up M's demon is to always make it, and unfortunately M by virtue of "its" residency in her, unhappy. We have to make it hard on the demon, and that means making it hard on M. My greatest sin here was to lie about the soup, insisting that it wasn't "creamy." I'm an idiot, totally patterned to always deny my deceit. What if I had just said, "Bingo, got me. But you ate it, right? You got through it, right? I'm an asshole, but that's my job." The biggest mistake today may not have been my being insensitive or myopic, but maybe that I missed the learning / growing / teaching moment. I could have made the case that she prevailed over a harder meal, that she notched another one on her belt in the ongoing war against her demon.

I want to make M happy, in the short and long term. I want to empathize with her struggle, and I want to know when she's fighting on my side of the battlefield. But I always have to keep my perspective on what are the best ways to help M win long term and how much is each tactic worth, either in making a dent in the demon or a dent in M's spirit. Within the battle of "state vs. weight," there seems to be a subset of "state" battle where I have to kill the demon by challenging her thinking, all the while bolstering her confidence and happiness to want to fight more on her own by my side.

The bottom line of this chapter is that there is no roadmap through this odyssey emotionally. No matter how well you know, or think you know your kid with an eating disorder, no matter how much you think you know how you will feel when dealing with your kid's situation…the layers of emotion within you that will be stung by this battle are endless. You will always get blindsided because you want some answers and truths to be just that, the answer, and the truth. But then they are not. What does happen with time, though, is this. The shelf life of the battles gets shorter. The days of silent treatment after a debate or fight become a day and then become an afternoon. Your inability to get it right, either by being too harsh on the demon and hurting your kids' feelings, or by going too soft on the demon to make your kid happy and then delay progress in recovery, will never go away. That dichotomy is the odyssey. That dichotomy is why every day is hard on you.

Chapter 15
Rigidity

One of the strongest weapons that an eating disorder will wield is rigid thinking. Rules, baby. Color inside the lines. No deviation, no evolution, no relaxing and going with the flow. And for many suffering with an eating disorder, this can be a manifestation of diagnosable OCD. Not just the punch line kind of habits or routines that we all joke about ("I'm getting my OCD on today to organize the pantry"), this is about an additional mental disorder that accelerates the evil game plan of eating disorders.

The rigidity, whether or not the child has OCD, will control everything about their eating habits. For example, they will have to eat the exact same meal plan today that they had yesterday, or they cannot repeat carbs for two consecutive meals, or since they hid food today, they will have to hide it again tomorrow. Rigid rules must be followed. So, part of your job in treating their "state of mind" is to break the rigid thinking. And for all the reasons this is hard to do, it is compounded when you are trying to get this kid on a regular eating schedule and get weight back on them. Routine is key to refeeding, but routine can also help accommodate rigidity.

So much of M's weight loss and resistance to recovery was not just her wanting to be thin. There were super strict and arbitrary rules that the demon put in place to limit any development or growth. And these rules were often fabricated in each situation to defend the demon's point of view. She would insist that protein portions could only be the size of three fingers. Nothing with white flour could be included as a carb. Morning snacks didn't exist in the real world. She could only eat in super small bowls, often transferring a regular bowl's worth into one. She would only eat with small crab forks. All of these, and many more, were the basis for her argumentative attitude when resisting. She would rest upon these rules as if they were self-evident.

We, in turn, specifically countered all that nonsense with exactly what she did not want. We hid all the small crab forks, we blocked the transfer from large bowls to small bowls, we plated white flour carbs for meals. And after a fight or two, M would ultimately scowl and abide and move on. And then, miraculously, that rule never came up again. This is another example of short-term pain for long term gain.

A small step in dealing with the rigid thinking is to deal with the asshole who is forcing this behavior. A classic way for patients and caregivers to refer to an eating disorder is to call it by the name it spells: ED. It's just simpler and saves everyone from saying "Anorexia Nervosa" or "Bulimia Nervosa" or "ARFID." Further, by naming a mental disorder, it separates that identity from the patient, which is important because the patient and the caregiver need to know and believe that the patient is not the demon, that the patient is not the one who wants to restrict or purge. There is a fantastic book by Jenni Schaefer called *Life Without Ed* in which she really brings this concept to life. And M, like many folks, took it one step further by customizing the name a bit. We call her demon "Edith." She sounds like a lovely woman, right?

We have taken the naming of M's disorder one step further by saying that M is not anxious or angry about a food, but instead we say that Edith is anxious or angry. M and Edith have separate feelings, M is not the one afraid of food. It's kind of like if you have a roommate that you hate and you want her to move out, so you just start talking about her in the third person right in front of her, yet you don't acknowledge her. Isolate, ostracize, and separate. M will loosen the rules and rigid thinking imposed on her by Edith by removing Edith from her identity.

To keep pushing this separation, we encourage M, in very small ways, to break away from any rules set by Edith. If she is still hungry at the end of the meal, she should have another bite or go get something else to eat. I KNOW, this is beyond Holy Grail stuff, but even one carrot is our goal. Show Edith that she had "more" and that "more" was ok. Rule broken. Additionally, if she wants to break up a meal by having her milk or juice an hour ahead because she's thirsty, that's great. And while food variety is great way of breaking rigid thinking, we are now only going after procedural issues. We want M to do things that Edith would not agree with. We want her to eat at times and places that

Edith would not approve of. And every time we break a rule and M feels ok about it, those behaviors will start to seem normal, and Edith will lose a little power.

Please know that for the most part, the best tactic against rigidity is persistence, there really is no magic fairy dust. But the persistence needs to be tempered with delicacy. Two days ago, we surprised M with a weigh-in she wasn't expecting. And while she had previously admitted to rigging her weight to show a higher number, she currently claimed that she stopped doing it. But lately, we were getting weight numbers week to week that made no sense.

Anyway, we pulled out the scale, she tried to protest, but even she realized that the more she protested the more she was admitting to not having prepped her deceit. So, the weight was about 6-8 pounds under where she needed to be, and way off from last week... even though she was eating everything. She stormed out and hid in her room. I waited a while and then texted her that I wanted to talk. Here a few quotes from the exchange.

"Nothing to talk about"

"Yes, please"

"It's only important to you guys"

"Please come and chat so we can move forward"

"No I don't wanna talk about weight gain, I've heard enough, your concern not a me concern"

"Please come and hear me"

"There's nothing to talk about, you're just gonna tell me I need to gain weight, I don't even hide food so I'm not doing anything wrong this time. This is literally just where my body has put me"

Here's my point about persistence and delicacy. I stayed super calm, super brief. I did not engage her debate points, did not respond to her complaints. I told her this was not about the past and that I was not going to scold her. She came downstairs from hiding in her room and leaned against the living room door frame with a posture that screamed "do NOT fuck with me." She started the conversation by saying that if I said one wrong word, she would leave. I stayed sitting on the floor, I paused before each sentence. My goal, and I had mapped this out, was to get her to agree to a slow change of food choices over time to get back to where she needed to be based on her doctor's assessment. All I could do was calmly ask her to hear my concerns and help me figure out some additions to her meal plan. But I also let her lead the conversation, let her speak, because the longer she talked, the more she stayed engaged.

At one point, she started to cry and blurted out how upset she was with herself. She was eating everything and not hiding or spitting up food, but she was failing to gain weight. And that in turn made her afraid of getting in trouble and being scolded, which is why she rigged her weight. Once these tears and admissions started rolling out, she softened up and dropped the anger. I told her I know how hard this is for her. I thanked her for helping me understand her perspective and her thinking. I then told her I'd like to go over some ideas about moving forward, and she agreed to having that conversation, but then said she needed to be alone… basically go get herself settled and calmed down.

Before bed that night, I asked her if we could walk Mason together early the next day, and she liked that. As we headed out on that walk the next morning, I again said very little, waiting for her to start the conversation. Within 15 minutes, she was talking about how hard the day before had been, how afraid she was of failing, and we had a nice chat together. By the end of the walk, we were able to agree that rigging the weigh-ins was not worth it for anyone, and she also agreed to an increase in both her lunch and snack with certain food substitutions. (Like I say throughout the book, density of fat and protein over bulk.)

Persistence in the face of rigidity is not easy, and at times it is hopeless. But staying super calm, knowing where the landmines are, avoiding a debate with the demon, and maybe even getting your kid to open up and ask for your help are the only tactics that worked for us. Empathy may have been the only lubricant that helped M open up, but not the cheesy "I'm here for you" kind. When M said how upset she was with herself for failing regardless of doing everything right, the lightbulb went on in my head. I agreed with her, told her she was doing a great job eating and trying new things, and I get it that she didn't want to fail or be judged or scolded. That helped her move a little in my direction when I said that I wanted to help her not fail and not feel scared about weigh-ins.

Like so many of the other events I have described in this book, the only way around rigid thinking is to break through it. You have to be persistent. Yes, it is such a pain in the ass to put out all these small fires but countering each rigid rule will be more small body blows to the demon that you are fighting. And as rigid thinking starts to soften up, you will have created an environment where new foods can be introduced, forbidden foods can finally rejoin the party, and healthy patterns of behavior can start to take root.

Chapter 16
In The Moment

As we have now lived through anorexia for over two and a half years, we are just starting to be a sounding board for other parents who are going through a similar struggle. I have said over and over in this book that eating disorders are so hidden in most communities, that I see very little of it and we know very few folks who are also suffering. Slowly, though, we have recently been introduced to a couple of families, through friends of friends, who are just starting their journey to hell and need someone to talk to.

As we counsel them on what the road ahead looks like, and as we give them advice on different treatment methods and refeeding techniques, we find that the most urgent questions we get from parents have to do with handling the initial conflicts when their kids refuse to eat. These parents have no idea what do to, and they are floored by the intensity of their kid's resistance to food. They are begging us to know the answer to the hardest question. "What do you do in that moment when your kid refuses to eat and runs away or screams at you? How do you force your kid to eat?"

These moments are nothing short of a crisis, because they bring together absolutely everything bad about eating disorders into one place in time: the mental anguish being wrought by an unseen demon, the hate and anger and rage of a child, the brutal conflict between parents and their kids, the desperate need to feed medicine to a sick child, the desperate need to de-escalate a volatile situation, and the blinding fear and terror of a parent who feels helpless and trapped.

As complex as this situation and this question are, the first answer is a simple one. You calm down, you buckle down, and you take your time. You are not fighting your kid; you are fighting a mental disorder who is trying to kill your kid. If you need to step back for a moment, then do it and collect yourself. But you are now in it for the long haul, and right now is step number one. You must marshal all of your calmness and your empathy and encourage your child to take small steps. The first step may be to get your kid to come out of the locked room or come back to the table. Be persistent, don't engage their arguments, and be supportive. Don't be dramatic or overly empathetic, but acknowledge that you know this is hard for them. Show them a distraction in the form of the TV, a TikTok video, a game, or some music. Anything to redirect or to break the tension. And keep being gently persistent about the fact that they have to start the meal and have a bite. Each bird-sized bite of the food they take is a win and allows that kid to take another.

This scenario is not a place for logical discourse or debates. Your child is scared and will try to use any argument that results in them not having to eat. They will ask how many calories are in the food, or if the portion is too big, or why is there a certain amount of protein or fat or carbohydrates. Your only response, along with being supportive and empathetic, is to say that the food is correct, and everything is fine. Say they can trust you, and that you know what you are doing. Do not answer their questions directly or offer up numbers or reasons. That will only drag out their resistance to eating and will create a longer debate that has no winner.

There is often the question of how much time do you allow this "moment" to drag out. Maybe set a 30-minute timer, and when that goes off, your child will have to supplement with Ensure for the calories that were not consumed. Or maybe the uneaten food on the plate is added to the next meal. Conversely, some parents will sit for two hours to enforce that all the food is eaten. That can be exhausting for both you and your kid, and it will then vastly shorten the time between meals…which means that you will have to start this whole shitstorm again in about an hour.

There is also the question of which works better, the carrot or the stick. Do you offer your kid a reward for eating, or do you threaten to take something away if your kid does not eat? That is a question that only you can answer, as only you know better which method could be more effective. I advocate for rewards in order to keep the short- and long-term energy positive. Plus, I did not want to take away anything that could help soothe my daughter in her downtime away from food, like her phone or the TV or seeing her friends. However, in extreme circumstances, be prepared to take the door off that kid's room so that they cannot hide food and they cannot exercise at night to burn calories; be prepared to remove the sheets from that kid's bed so they cannot find comfort in their room when trying to hide from you; be prepared even to call the cops on that kid when they threaten to or actually commit harmful violence against themselves or you.

This pattern of your kid resisting food and fighting you, while you encourage and continue to feed, will repeat itself multiple times a day, for days at a time, and then for weeks at a time. But the more you go through this routine, the easier it will become for both you and your child. The more you do it, the more comfortable you will be at engaging this crazy behavior. And the more you do it, the quicker the demon will see that you are serious and that this child it is inhabiting may not be for sale.

By jumping in one hundred percent on each "moment" and engaging the demon, regardless of how you decide to time and / or supplement, and whether you decide to reward or punish, you are setting the stage for long-term treatment. Recovery is made up of five to seven meals a day, seven days a week, on into the future. There are no "cheat" days. But the more you engage these moments early on, the stronger you will be in the long run.

Chapter 17

This is Not an Exit

We are approaching the three-year anniversary of M being admitted to the hospital for the first time and are way down the road of doing FBT at home. We have seen entire years go by, all the holidays and all the seasons cycle through while battling the demon. We spent the entirety of COVID-19 at home with a teenage girl who was going through all the normal remote shit, but who also had to think about calories all day in her room. Our life's "new normal" is feeding M. I almost cannot remember looking at M and not seeing Anorexia, not worrying about her weight, and not being scared of what our next conflict will be about. But at the same time, since that is our only normal and our only reality now, there is some comfort in looking back and seeing how far we have come.

We are well into phase three of FBT. Phase one is where we parents shop, prep, and plate all food. Phase two is collaborative, in that M started taking responsibility for part of her own food choices and prep. As I have discussed before, this second phase was where M started showing her disorder that she was willing to join the fight against it and provide to herself the medicine that would kill it. Phase three is now where the training wheels come off the bike, where the water wings on the arms of a child in the pool are removed. She has to march forward on her own and take control of her recovery. We can only hope that all the training we went through will yield the right skills and habits for her. And still, I am very close by, at all times, to show her that there is support.

This separation of us from M, and of M from Edith, is a long and slow process. M plans out all of her meals, and shops for the brands she wants. She preps and eats every meal that she is supposed to, with no prompting from me. She eats out with friends more and more, sometimes without seeing the menu ahead of time. But she always has a sense of hesitancy, and she admits that she wants me around for some meals. She admits that she still needs me there to, in her mind, enforce that she follows through. She sees and wants recovery, in the form of freedom from rigid eating patterns and with a license to indulge new foods. And while this last step may not be hardest in her journey, it is definitely the step that will take the longest amount of time.

Her "state" of mind has gained so much strength, so much maturity, so much clarity. She is sober and separated from wanting to restrict, and she is not angry at the world. She knows she needs to eat, she knows she has to gain weight, she knows that she does not ever again want to be malnourished and vastly underweight. I love this M, this lucid and learned veteran of a horrible war, who cracks wise about her "issues" and how she has probably ruined the lives of many therapists. But all this "state" largess, all of this clarity of mind, is still at risk of having the drain unplugged below it if she doesn't maintain a healthy "weight." She still has to pick up another 4-5 pounds, and that is currently an epic battle each day as she is in charge of each ingredient, and each portion, of each meal. All the talk and intention are there, but the actual calorie intake that is needed does not always happen.

The best analogy to where we are right now with M is a baseball game. One team (us) got way behind early on, they went through most of their pitchers, and they also lost some key players to injury. Through grit and hard work, they evened the score and found a way to temper the bats of the stronger team (Edith). But now they have to slog through the eternity of the middle innings of the game, pitch by pitch, hoping to score a run or two in order to get to the end of the ninth inning and be ahead and call it a win. We are living our life pitch by pitch, meal by meal, weekly weigh-in by weekly weigh-in, hoping that M inches up to her target weight while never letting the demon regain control of her, all before she goes off to college.

Tina and I are starting to let our shoulders down a little bit, are starting to feel some of the fear and anxiety of the last couple of years wash off our backs. It is so tempting to wake up one day and say, "Ok, M, you're good. Just keep eating this way, we'll stop seeing Dr. Aspen, and you'll be good. Your path seems straight, and you seem to have beaten back the demon." But we know that we cannot let up our vigilance, we know that we must be mindful of course-correcting

M's behavior and measuring her status. Just the other day, for example, we were talking to M about how well she was eating and how we thought we saw that she was relaxing about rigid eating patterns. She laughingly scoffed at us and said, "It's not like I look at the clock and say, 'Wow, it's 3:00, I should have a snack'. No, I'm anorexic, I'm in my room at 1:28 and thinking, 'Only 92 minutes to snack'." Eating disorders check into your kids' brains and ask for the long-term lease. They are not short-term tenants. It is exhausting to be the food police and the demon SWAT team every day for years, but if you have gotten as far as we have, you cannot let up. This is tiring, but it is actually so much easier than it has ever been. Now starts the slower and less intense march, but it is still a march.

And here is another way that I have come to view this march. I may be tired, but most families, if not all, go through trauma. They go through sickness, or suffering, or struggle. Some families face death, others battle substance abuse or physical abuse or sexual abuse. Some families are estranged from each other; some families have no family at all. When I have opened up to other people and parents about our experience with anorexia, most respond with a knowing look and a story about what their family has gone through. There is no measuring stick or comparison chart between us, there is only a common understanding of knowing what it is like to go down a road to hell with family. Fear and anger and anxiety and dread and depression are shared experiences, and just making myself realize that fact helps me know I am not alone. I've got my shit, and so does everyone else.

I truly believe that M will be free from the demon one day and it will be for good. Having that horizon, that hope, and that knowledge helps each day be ok for me. Having the perspective that the end could arrive, and I could chalk up the win, brings me peace. Not everyone with a struggling child can say that, because eating disorders can be so elusive and relentless and deadly. But I have my hope and I have my battle scars and I have my daughter. I also have nowhere to go but forward toward the end.

Acknowledgments

Tina, you showed me how to treat her. There is no one other than you that I could or would have gone through this with. Ronin, you're a great brother and wonderful son and you opened our eyes. We love you very much. Dr. Sue Knight, you saved M's life. Go Bears! Dr. Vandana Aspen: You, are the gold standard. Stanford Children's Health Eating Disorder Program, this lifelong Cal family owes you more than we can ever pay. Dr Dipti Bhakta, thank you for helping to soften the blow. Famdamnly, what can I say? You rallied around M, you rallied around us, you watched and listened and loved. That's all we needed. Eric, I never knew what you went through. I still wish I didn't. E.R.M., you showed me that strength and time could result in recovery. Thank you. Ella, what you did for M when no one was looking showed me how much character and love you have. Tom, thanks for always asking. Frannie & Mason, thanks for always listening. Lynne, your title may have been "tutor," but you were the best friend M could have had. David Solomon, I so appreciated your help in making a lot of little things work out. Rad, you brought clarity in the middle of chaos, and you got M through math.

The Monterey County Sheriff's Department and City of Carmel by the Sea Police Department, thank you for literally answering the call when I was at my lowest. Contra Costa County Sheriff's Department, you were our BAM moment. You were awesome. Sorry for what M said to you. Richard Barnes, you said it all in one sentence. Dr. Dana Rygg, Dr. Alexandra Tee, Aimee Paulson, Claudine Cho, Wendy Sterling, Kirsten Graves, Dr. Sara Buckelew: you all gave me invaluable insight and information, please keep helping people. Dr. Kerri Turner, your initial guidance was critical. Kelly Way, everyone needs a good attorney, and that you are. Donger, you affirmed my voice and cleaned up my crap. To all my old friends, you are the best friends. To everyone at the butcher counter at Lunardi's, you are my happy place.

Additional gratitude to Jen Hemmer, Leslie and Dave Morris, Kathy Oxley, Julian Brooks, Julia Brochstein, Heather Hohl, Val Sherer and Jeff Long. And a special thanks to The Men of FEAST for all the honesty and support.

To anyone who is not mentioned here, please know it was an oversight and not an omission. There was an overwhelming amount of community and family who were a part of our journey, and my mind doesn't always remember all it should. Therefore, thank you to all!

About The Author

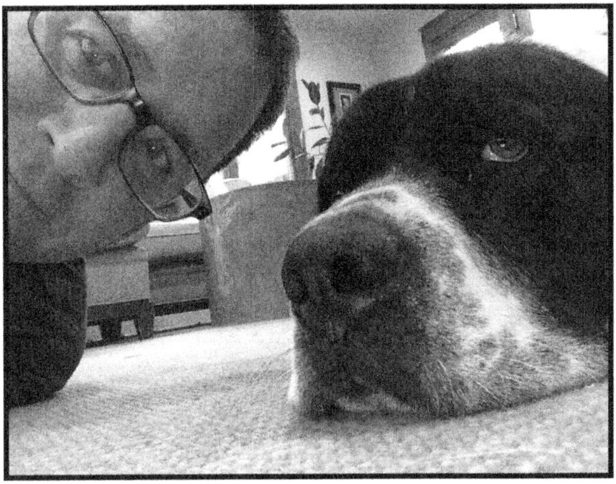

Kevin Olmsted is a pretty average suburban Dad living in Northern California. He is a proud graduate of UC Berkeley, a 23-year veteran of the wine business and is a former Certified Sommelier. He loves to cook too much food for friends, he's a terrible golfer, and he talks to his dogs five times more that he talks to most humans.

Along with writing this book, Kevin speaks to parent groups in his community and around Northern California about eating disorders. His goal is the be "that person" who wasn't there for him when M first got sick. He wants to be a first call, a resource, an answer to a question for any parent who first encounters a child's eating disorder. Please learn more about Kevin's and M's journey by visiting their website Scareddadfeeding.com.

This is Kevin's first book, and as long as M continues her recovery, it should be his last.

Printed in Great Britain
by Amazon

50979594R00089